Healing Tonics

101 Herbal Concoctions to Increase
Energy, Boost Immunity, Enhance
Memory, Ease Digestion, and
Support Daily Health and Wellness

JEANINE POLLAK

STOREY
BOOKS

The mission of Storey Publishing is to serve our customers by publishing practical information that encourages personal independence in harmony with the environment.

Edited by Deborah Balmuth and Robin Catalano
Cover design by Meredith Maker
Text design and production by Erin Lincourt
Cover and interior photographs by Giles Prett except individual herbalists and photographs on pages 31, 43, 53, 63, 71, 79, 87, and 93 © Martin Wall; pages 16, 45, 50, 99, and 119 by A. Blake Gardner; page 117 by Cynthia McFarland; pages 56, 74, 95, and 116 © Jeff Burke and Lorraine Triolo for Artville; and pages 100, 101, 125, and 134 © PhotoDisk, Inc.
Indexed by Nan Badgett, Word•a•bil•i•ty

The information in this book is true and complete to the best of our knowledge. All recommendations are made without guarantee on the part of the author or Storey Publishing. The author and publisher disclaim any liability in connection with the use of this information. For additional information please contact Storey Books, 210 MASS MoCA Way, North Adams, MA 01247.

Storey books are available for special premium and promotional uses and for customized editions. For further information, please call Storey's Custom Publishing Department at 1-800-793-9396.

Printed in Canada by Transcontinental Printing
10 9 8 7

Library of Congress Cataloging-in-Publication Data

Pollak, Jeanine, 1957-
    Healing tonics : 101 herbal concoctions to increase energy, boost immunity, enhance memory, ease digestion, and support daily health and wellness / Jeanine Faith Pollak.
        p.   cm.
     ISBN 1-58017-240-7 (pbk. : alk. paper)
     1. Tonics (Medicinal preparations) 2. Herbs—Therapeutic use. I. Title.
RM239.P65 2000
615'.321—dc21
                                                 99-089105
                                               CIP

Contents

Herbalist Profiles

Dedication

In loving memory of my father, Victor Pollak, whose sense of humor and love of gardening continue to shape and inspire me.

Acknowledgments

Many thanks to my fabulous editors at Storey, Deborah Balmuth and Robin Catalano. Your creative insight and helpful suggestions have facilitated each important phase of this book. It has been a pleasure working with you both. And thanks again for bringing me out to Massachusetts in June of 1999. It was great fun brainstorming and planning *Healing Tonics* with the staff at Storey, and taking the time to explore the local wild plants and countryside.

I would also like to thank my sweetheart, Richard Turner, for encouraging me to stop throwing so many dinner parties and start writing down my recipes, and for humoring me during my early computer phobia.

Many thanks also to Mary Nosse ("Proud Mary") for your unfaltering organizational skills and for helping contact the guest herbalists who contributed to this book. Your assistance in both my classes and with the manuscript has been absolutely essential this past year!

Thanks to Judith Marks, for sitting so calmly with me the day this manuscript was due, and helping format it all so effortlessly.

Heartfelt thanks to all my incredible students over the past 23 years. It was in your presence that many of these recipes were born, often spontaneously, in the midst of my teaching. Thank you for your interest in my work, and for all the amazing meals, hikes, travels, and adventures we've shared over the years. It is a blessing to be able to do what I love, and continually meet and interact with great people along the way! To your health, happiness, and vitality — enjoy these recipes and always keep your connection to the plants and the places where they grow.

Introduction to Healing Tonics

the concept of using tonics is as old as herbalism itself. To tonify is to nourish, strengthen, and increase the vitality of the body and internal organs. Rather than waiting until you get sick and then trying to fix the problem, tonics offer the proactive step of strengthening and building up the body.

Herbs have the profound ability to promote health, and herbal tonics have the unique ability to nourish, fortify, and balance the major organ systems of the body. Tonic herbs are herbs that are nutritive and vitamin- and mineral-rich. These plants are usually appropriate for long-term use, since they work slowly and steadily to strengthen the body and its organ systems. Some tonic herbs have an affect on specific organ systems through their nutritive action, while others have certain constituents that strengthen and tonify. For instance, hawthorn contains flavonoids that fortify the heart and enhance circulation, and ginseng's saponin glycosides tonify the adrenals.

To enhance the immune system, build the blood, tone the digestive tract, balance the hormones, strengthen the heart, and nourish the nerves, I offer you this colorful and flavorful collection of recipes for optimal wellness.

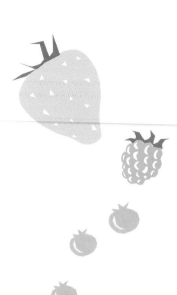

Nourishing the Body, Mind, and Soul

Some of my earliest childhood memories revolve around the kitchen. I spent many a day experimenting with tastes and textures, studying recipes and then throwing them aside, deciding that it was easier to make them up along the way.

By the time I was a teenager, most of my friends' kitchens were quite familiar to me. I loved cooking and baking anywhere, anytime. My mom used to tease me and warn me not to assume that my friends would welcome my mad extravaganzas in their kitchens.

When I was 18, I went to my first springtime herb retreat in northern California. The very first class I attended was an herb walk, and it changed my life. Suddenly, all these little green things growing in the ground had names, unique histories and uses, and the potential to be enjoyed as food and transformed into medicine. A new world of qualities, textures, and tastes opened up. I was fascinated and inspired, and I couldn't stop looking at the ground, so curious about all these new little green friends. I began a love affair with the world of plants that has captivated me ever since.

I began gathering and concocting with wild plants almost immediately. Soon I was teaching others about plants. I must thank my open-minded college roommates for trustingly eating all the wild greens I prepared that first year. As a matter of course, I started making tinctures and salves. Then began a new phase, the creative process of formulating herbal products. This was my goal: The formulas must work like a charm and also taste so good that people would want to take them, even crave them and enjoy them. Soon bottles full of potions and tonics lined my kitchen and cupboards. So began the great experiments of a young herbalist-wanna-be.

As my herbal skills increased, so did the demand for my newly created herbal formulas. Neighbors and friends appeared with specific requests . . . and so my repertoire of products kept expanding. Often I would make something new, and suddenly several people in my life would need that exact herbal formula.

Well, here it is 23 years later, and now there are bottles full of potions all over my house, on every shelf, lining every available corner. (I knew I had to do something last year, when one by one, all the shelves in my kitchen cupboard fell down from the weight of too many bottles!) The love of concocting delicious formulas still runs in my blood, and, like anyone who gets struck by the creative urge, I delight in the process of bringing these recipes to fruition.

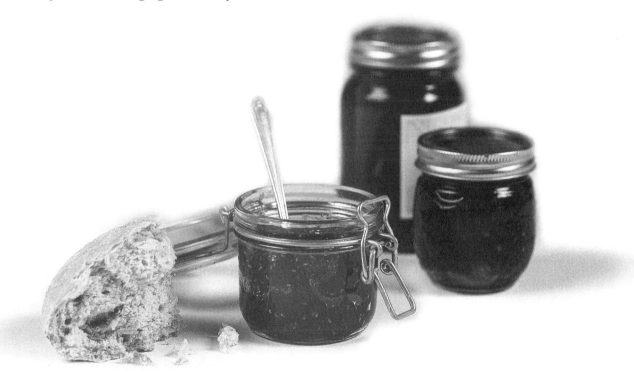

Empower Yourself with Herbal Medicines

It seems that there's an increasing interest in getting to know herbs and learning to use them properly. The concept of tonics is a timely one: Enhancing natural resistance, building strength and vitality, and increasing energy are all worthy goals in personal health care.

But beyond that aim, have fun, take time, and enjoy the process of making your own special concoctions. The extracting and transforming of individual ingredients into delicious tonics is quite rewarding, and there's a world of creative possibilities awaiting you. Ultimately, it's empowering to learn to make your own unique and useful herbal formulas.

With my love of fresh plants, hiking, spending time in gardens and in kitchens, and creating yummy things to eat and drink, it seems this is a most appropriate book to have written. May your taste buds and creative process lead you down a most enjoyable path of self-nourishment and increased health and well-being.

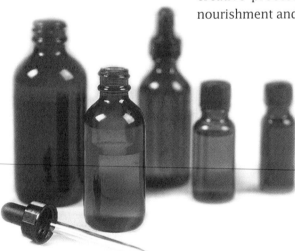

Making Teas, Tinctures, Cordials & Elixirs

This chapter offers a wealth of information about making your own herbal teas, tinctures, and cordials. There is an art and a science to making well-balanced, effective, and tasty formulas, and this book is dedicated to teaching you how to make such formulas in your own kitchen. The process of making your own herbal products is exciting, rewarding, and ultimately empowering. I hope you will be inspired to try the recipes presented later in the book, and then reap the benefits.

Getting Organized:
The Tools of the Trade

The supplies that you'll need to make your own tonics are fairly basic, and you'll probably find that you have most of them in your kitchen already. For the few things that you may need to purchase, your local grocery, hardware, and kitchen supply stores will probably suffice. If you need to order any particular items that are hard to find, check Resources for more options.

Kitchenware Basics

I'm a firm believer in having lots of kitchen basics around — clean glass jars with lids, labels, cheesecloth, strainers, colanders, and so on. That way, if the urge to make a recipe hits, you'll be prepared! Besides, who wants to go shopping when you could be out gathering fresh herbs from which to create an absolutely stunning, mouth-watering, once-in-a-lifetime concoction?

The following list is general, but it gives a good idea of the kinds of supplies that are helpful in making herbal recipes.

Glass Jars

A variety of clean glass jars is useful for storing dry herbs and steeping and storing your tinctures and cordials. Most markets and hardware stores sell canning jars by the case. I find the 8-ounce, 16-ounce, 32-ounce, and 64-ounce sizes most useful.

Empty glass jars from jams, jellies, and peanut butter are all useful, too; just be sure to wash and dry them thoroughly. The odors tend to linger in jars that originally contained pickles, garlic, or onions. The jars themselves can usually be washed out and deodorized, but the lids tend to hold on to smells for a long time. It's best not to use these jars to make or store your herbal products.

Lids

Lids for your jars should be clean and odor-free; avoid reusing lids that have lingering odors of garlic, tomato sauce, or pickled vegetables. If you must, at least cover the opening of the jar with plastic wrap before securing the lid. Plastic wrap isn't usually recommended, but it does help with odor control and can prevent the rusting of jar lids. You can also purchase new canning jar lids in most supermarkets or hardware stores.

Labels

Label the bottles of everything you make! You will be tempted to make wonderful, unlabeled concoctions. Your mind will swear that you'll remember everything. From the years of discovering many a jar of unlabeled tincture, I will say only this: Cultivate good habits early on.

A good label should have:

❋ The name of the product
❋ The date you started making the product
❋ A list of all ingredients, including the type of menstruum (liquid or solvent)
❋ Any special cautions or considerations

While any old label will do for tinctures-in-progress, you may want to purchase or make some festive labels for your final products. Check local herb, card, and stationery stores for creative labels.

Straining Supplies

Straining materials are also a necessity for tonic making.

Cheesecloth and fine nylon mesh, such as 1-gallon paint-straining bags, work great to strain your products. Both types of straining materials are available at most hardware stores. Cheesecloth is also available at most grocery stores. If using cheesecloth, double or triple the layers so that you trap as many of the finer particles as possible.

Colanders and strainers, which you probably already have, are a helpful addition to your kitchen "pharmacy." A regular-sized colander and a few various-sized strainers are useful. Make sure you purchase some fine-mesh strainers, which are readily available at most kitchen supply stores.

Wooden spoons and spatulas are good for stirring and scraping things out of jars.

Pots and Pans

Most people already have a diversity of cookware in their kitchens. The best kinds of cookware to use include glass, stainless steel, and coated enamel. Avoid using aluminum, as it reacts with herbs and foods and may leach into your products. As for cast iron, I use it to cook with but not for making teas, syrups, or conserves, as it also reacts with herbs and fruits.

Bottles

Amber glass dropper bottles and smaller jars are useful for packaging, storing, or carting around small amounts of your tinctures and cordials. There are also a lot of beautiful colored glass bottles available these days, and they add a nice touch to the packaging of products. Check your local herb or natural foods store, as well as local gourmet and kitchen stores. Many companies also sell bottles via mail order (see Resources for more information).

Blenders and Grinders

A normal kitchen blender works well to whip up fresh tinctures, smoothies, and more. The common electric coffee grinders work well for grinding most dry herbs into powders. I recommend getting a separate grinder just for herbs; otherwise, you may find that your fresh ground coffee has some unusual flavors!

One trick for cleaning out grinders is to wipe all the herb powder out and then clean under the blades with a cotton swab. Moisten a clean cloth with a little brandy or vodka, and then wipe out the inside of the grinder. This cleans up any resinous or aromatic residue and leaves the grinder shiny clean. Wash the lid in hot soapy water, rinse well, dry, and you'll be ready to go.

Funnels or Paper Cups

These two items are useful when transferring tinctures and syrups to smaller, thin-necked bottles. Small funnels work well, or you can pour the liquid into a paper cup, squeeze it to form a pouring spout, and then pour the liquid from the cup into the bottle.

Herb Press

If you find yourself making lots of tinctures and other products that need straining, you may want to purchase an herb press. This press works by squeezing the herbal material against a finely perforated stainless steel canister; the resulting liquid then seeps through a series of canisters and tubes into a clean bowl at the bottom. Herb presses vary in style and size, but, generally, a small wine press will do the trick. If you have strong hands and like to get right into the straining process, a press isn't really necessary. Good-quality herb presses can be ordered through your local beer and wine supply stores.

Grinding Hard Roots

Some of the very hard Chinese roots, such as ginseng and dong quai, may have to be broken up into little pieces before grinding. Break a root by wrapping it loosely in a dishtowel, placing the wrapped root on a cutting board, and hitting it hard with a heavy frying pan or a hammer.

How to Make Herbal Medicines

If you are just beginning to learn about herbs, you might find yourself standing in the aisles of an herb store, staring, overwhelmed, at the shelves. Bulk teas? You mean they don't all come in nice dry, dependable little tea bags? How much bulk herb do I use with how much water? When do I boil and when do I steep?

And what about tinctures? Why do we pour alcohol all over something as healthy as herbs anyway? And those funny things called cordials — aren't they something that elderly English ladies used to sip in the late afternoon? (Probably so, as smart as these ladies were.)

This section provides concise steps for making herbal teas, tinctures, and cordials. You will find references to this section in the recipes throughout the book. Look here whenever you need more detailed information on all aspects of herbal preparations.

Tea

All tea is not created equal. Like anything good in life, it takes a bit of knowledge, the proper tools, and a dash or two of creativity to make a truly fine herbal brew. Read over these basics of the creative art of truly fine tea making.

To get started, you'll need:

❋ A good glass teapot, or a stainless steel, enamel, or glass French press. (I am partial to glass teapots, which allow me to enjoy all the colorful visuals of the herbs and flowers.)

❋ A fine-mesh strainer. Forget those silly little metal tea balls. They are an insult to any real tea-making experience. Herbs like to float in water, unencumbered.

❋ Some basic background on individual herbs and their properties. See A Materia Medica of Tonic Herbs for detailed information on different herbs and their properties.

Choosing and Measuring Herbs

Dry herbs will never equal fresh when it comes to nutritive value, vitality, flavor, and texture. Learning to grow or wildcraft (gather fresh wild herbs from their natural habitat) edible herbs and flowers will greatly enhance your tea-making experience. When wildcrafting, keep in mind these three important principles: identify plants properly; choose a clean, toxin-free environment from which to pick plants; and *never* overharvest wild plants from their natural environments. If growing or wildcrafting isn't possible for you, then check your local herb stores for the best quality, "freshest" dried herbs. Buy organic whenever possible, and support local ethical wildcrafters in your area.

The simplest way to measure herbs for recipes is in "parts." In this way, the measurement is determined in relation to the other ingredients in the formula. A part can be any unit of measurement, such as teaspoons, tablespoons, or cups, but each part should be used consistently throughout the formula. Thus, if a recipe calls for 3 parts passionflower, 1 part lemon balm, and 2 parts oats, you might use 3 teaspoons passionflower, 1 teaspoon lemon balm, and 2 teaspoons oats.

Since most herbalists seem incapable of measuring anything with an actual measuring cup, we get very good at measuring by the "handful" (a handful can also represent a part). If you happen to be one of those very precise people, the general guideline for teas is 1 ounce of dried herb to 1 quart of boiling water. One ounce of dried herb occupies somewhere between ¼ and 1 cup, depending on the density of the herb. For lightweight dry herbs, such as mullein, red clover blossoms, and wild oat, 1 ounce equals approximately 1 cup of the herb. For dry roots and seeds, such as dandelion root, burdock root, and rose hips or fennel, 1 ounce equals approximately ¼–½ cup. For fresh herbs, use roughly twice the amount as dried, generally, ½–1 cup of fresh herbs per quart of boiling water.

The proportion of herbs to water will vary a bit with the strength, density, and taste of the herbs. If, for instance, you are working with some very bitter herbs, you may want to lighten up just a wee bit, lest you scare your poor, unsuspecting taste buds or horrify your guests. If working with bulk herbs is new to you, bring a standard 8-ounce measuring cup with you to your nearest herb store. Weigh out 1 ounce of a few different herbs, pour them into your measuring cup, and see for yourself how different 1 ounce of red clover blossoms is from 1 ounce of rose hips or dandelion root. This is a great visual and tactile learning experience for novice tea makers.

How to Make and Use an Infusion (from Leaves and Flowers)

A type of herbal tea, an infusion is made by steeping the herb's leaves and flowers in boiling water.

To make:

1. Measure out 1–2 ounces (about ½–1 cup) of dried herbs per quart of boiling water. If using fresh herbs, double the amount of plant material. Combine the herbs in a pot.

2. Pour 1 quart of boiling water over the herbs. Stir well, cover, and steep for 15–20 minutes.

3. Strain, and sweeten lightly with honey if desired.

To use: Enjoy 1–4 cups of infusion per day, depending on the formula and the condition being treated. Generally, 1–2 cups per day are used for a tonic dose, while 3–4 cups per day are drunk for a medicinal dose.

How to Make and Use a Decoction (from Roots, Bark, and Berries)

Like an infusion, a decoction is a type of herbal tea. This preparation is made by boiling the roots, bark, or berries of an herb.

To make:

1. Measure out approximately 1 ounce (½ cup) of dried herbs per quart of boiling water. If using fresh herbs, double the amount of herbs. Combine all herbs in a pot.

2. Pour 1 quart of water over the herbs. Bring to a boil.

3. Stir well, cover, and reduce heat to a simmer.

4. Simmer for 15–45 minutes, depending on the strength and flavor of the herbs you are using. For very hard and woody herbs, especially Chinese roots such as ginseng and astragalus, simmer 1–2 hours.

5. Strain, and sweeten lightly with honey if desired.

To use: Enjoy 1–4 cups of decoction per day, depending on the formula and the treatment. Generally, drink 1–2 cups per day for a tonic dose, or 3–4 cups per day for a medicinal dose.

What do you do when working with those really nasty-tasting herbs? To save yourself a lot of grimacing and taste-bud misery, try aromatic carminatives; they go a long way as "flavor savers" when added to bitter formulas. Plus, most aromatic carminatives benefit the stomach and lungs, so they're great additions to formulas of this nature. Examples of this type of herb are anise, cardamom, cinnamon, fennel, ginger, lemon balm, lemon verbena, orange (fruit and peel), and mints.

As you get the know the tastes and qualities of different herbs, you'll be able to adjust for both the strength of the herb and its flavor.

Tinctures

Tinctures are a potent and convenient way of taking herbs. Tinctures are concentrated, convenient to take, and easily absorbed. They are also very stable and can be stored for years at a time.

Alcohol, such as brandy or vodka, is commonly used as a *menstruum* for the making of tinctures. The menstruum is the liquid, or solvent, used to extract the herbs. Alcohol is a strong polar solvent, which means that it has the ability to pull the medicinal constituents out of herbs quite easily. Alcohol also acts as a good preservative for the finished tincture. Because tinctures are taken in very small amounts per dose, the amount of alcohol is minimal. Note: *Isopropyl or "rubbing" alcohol should never be used for internal preparations.* See the caution on page 18 for more information.

But for those who wish to make nonalcohol-based tinctures, try using apple cider vinegar or vegetable glycerin — a naturally sweet and syrupy by-product of olive oil extraction — in place of the alcohol. You can even mix half cider vinegar and half vegetable glycerin for a sweeter-tasting base. While neither of these solvents is quite as strong as alcohol, they both offer good alternatives to alcohol-based tinctures. Glycerin is generally considered a stronger solvent than vinegar. You can purchase vegetable glycerin in most herb or natural foods stores (see Resources for direct ordering). Glycerin-based tinctures are also known as glycerites.

How to Make and Use a Tincture
To make:

1. Wash and chop fresh herbs, removing any woody stems, or grind the dry herbs (do not wash dry herbs) into a fine powder.

2. Place all ingredients in a widemouthed glass jar. If using fresh herbs, cover with twice as much vodka or brandy. If using dried herbs, cover with 3 times as much vodka or brandy. You can also blend the herbs and alcohol in a blender until smooth to help the alcohol extract even more from the herbs. Then transfer the blended liquid to a glass jar. To prevent molding, make sure that there are no air bubbles in the liquid and that the liquid covers the top of the plant material.

If using glycerin to tincture dry herbs, use ⅔ cup glycerin and ⅓ cup water for every cup of base you need. If tincturing fresh herbs, use the glycerin undiluted, since fresh herbs have plenty of water in them. Your goal is to cover the herbs with 2 to 3 times as much glycerin base. For instance, if you're using 1 cup of fresh herbs, cover with 2 cups of undiluted glycerin.

3. Cover the jar, and store at room temperature away from direct light and heat. Shake daily for 2–4 weeks.

4. Strain through a fine nylon or muslin bag or cheesecloth (fine-mesh nylon 1-gallon paint-straining bags work great), squeezing as much liquid as possible out of the herbs.

5. Compost the herbs and rebottle the tincture. When stored in a cool, dark place, the tincture will last indefinitely.

To use: Take 1–2 droppersful (¼–½ teaspoon) once a day as a preventive tonic, or 1–2 droppersful 3–5 times per day as an acute remedy for a specific condition. Take tincture in a small amount of water, tea, or juice.

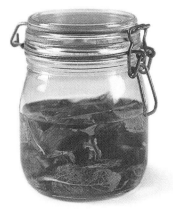

Using Combinations of Fresh and Dried Herbs

If you're making a tincture with some fresh and some dry herbs and roots:

1. Chop or mince the fresh herbs/roots. Grind the dry herbs/roots in a coffee grinder.
2. Place all herbs in a blender. Cover with 3 times as much brandy or vodka, and blend until smooth.
3. Pour the liquid into a glass jar and cover tightly. Store at room temperature away from direct light and heat. Shake daily for 2–4 weeks.
4. Strain through a fine nylon or muslin bag or cheese-cloth, squeezing as much liquid as possible out of the herbs.
5. Compost the herbs and rebottle the tincture. Store in a cool, dark place.

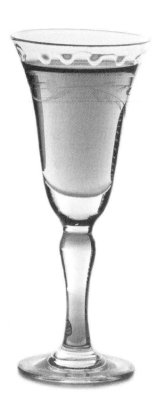

Cordials and Elixirs

Cordials and elixirs are interchangeable terms for lightly sweetened, delicious, tincture-based medicinal herbal tonics. They often contain herbs, fruits, and berries for flavor, color, and nutritional value. Seasonal organic fresh fruits and berries from your local area add a wonderful dimension to your herbal-product making. Excellent fresh fruits to include in your cordials are:

- ✳ Apricots
- ✳ Blackberries
- ✳ Blueberries
- ✳ Nectarines
- ✳ Oranges or tangerines
- ✳ Peaches
- ✳ Pears
- ✳ Persimmons
- ✳ Plums
- ✳ Raspberries
- ✳ Rose hips
- ✳ Strawberries

To make a cordial or elixir, you'll first need to make a tincture. After the tincture is strained, lightly sweeten it. I generally use ¼–½ cup maple syrup, honey, or molasses per quart of cordial or elixir. While traditional cordials and elixirs are alcohol-based, you can use glycerin as an alternate menstruum. Because glycerin is naturally sweet, you do not need additional sweeteners. Technically, glycerin-based tinctures are glycerites, but some of them are so delicious and festive that I refer to them as cordials or elixirs.

Note: *Isopropyl or "rubbing" alcohol should never be used for internal preparations.* See the caution on page 18 for more information.

How to Make a Cordial

1. Chop the fresh herbs, fruits, and berries. Grind dry herbs.

2. Place all ingredients in a widemouthed glass jar. Cover with 3 times as much vodka or brandy.

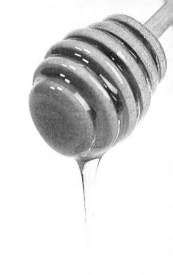

3. Cover the jar; store at room temperature away from direct light and heat. Shake daily for 2–4 weeks.

4. Strain well, squeezing as much liquid as possible out of the steeped herbs.

5. Compost the herbs and rebottle the cordial. Sweeten cordial lightly with ¼–½ cup honey, molasses, or maple syrup per quart of cordial.

Solvents and Solubilities of Alcohol

Questions always come up about solvents and solubilities of alcohol with regard to tincture making. Here are a few simple rules and guidelines:

Golden Rule #1: The "proof" of an alcohol is twice as strong as the percentage. Therefore:

* ❋ 80 proof = 40 percent alcohol
* ❋ 100 proof = 50 percent alcohol
* ❋ 150 proof = 75 percent alcohol
* ❋ 190 proof = 95 percent alcohol (yee ha!!!)

Golden Rule #2: For most tincture making, 80-proof alcohol, such as brandy or vodka, will be sufficient. For almost all tonic, cordial, and elixir formulas, either brandy or vodka (80 proof) will do just fine.

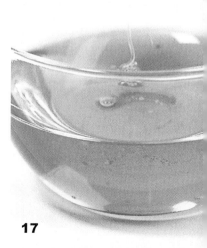

Locating the Right Proof Alcohol

Check your local liquor store. In California, the highest percentage alcohol available is about 75 percent (150 proof), under the brand name Everclear. In Arizona, Connecticut, Kentucky, New Mexico, Missouri, and several other states, true 190-proof ethanol (95 percent pure grain alcohol) is available. You can also mail-order pure food-grade ethanol (see Resources for more information).

Golden Rule #3: Brandy is a bit more flavorful and a tad sweeter than vodka, and it lends itself nicely to tonic formulas, cordials and elixirs, and bitter formulas.

Golden Rule #4: When working with resinous herbs — such as calendula, chaparral, grindelia, yerba santa, lavender, rosemary, and sage (the latter three herbs are rich in essential oils, which makes them rather sticky) — a higher percentage of alcohol is needed to properly extract all of the herb's medicinal properties. Generally, 60–75 percent alcohol is a good percentage to shoot for. When tincturing usnea or milk thistle seed, a higher percentage of alcohol is also needed (about 70–90 percent). These two herbs are not resinous, but because of their unique chemistry they require a higher strength alcohol to extract completely.

Golden Rule #5: How do you dilute pure ethanol to the percentage you want? Let's say you purchase some pure food-grade ethanol that is 190 proof, or 95 percent alcohol, and you want it diluted to 60 percent to make a tincture. Simply add ⅓ cup pure distilled water to every ⅔ cup ethanol, and you will have approximately a 60 percent base to work with. If you are starting with 95 percent ethanol and wish to dilute it down to about 50 percent, mix equal parts ethanol and distilled water. It's that simple!

Important Safety Precaution

Never use isopropyl ("rubbing") alcohol or denatured alcohol in your tinctures or cordials; these alcohols are deadly poisons. Use only good-quality brandy, vodka, or certified food-grade ethanol for tincture and cordial making.

Vitality Boosters & Energy Enhancers

What an appropriate place to start the recipe section of a book on tonics! The following recipes are deep, rich, colorful brews that are full of nourishing qualities. Feeling a little overworked, stressed, or just plain tuckered out? Perhaps "lackluster" is your new middle name? This chapter is for you!

Many of these recipes are food- and tea-based and can be prepared "on the spot," as needed. Other recipes are cordials and tonics, which need longer steeping times. It's nice to start making these longer-steeped tonics in late summer to early autumn, so they'll be ready to enjoy during the colder winter months.

Whichever recipes you decide to try, know that you are doing something truly energy-building and life-enhancing for yourself. Enjoy; this is quite an exotic assortment of vitality-boosting delights!

10 Treasures Vitality Tonic

*This is a deeply tonifying
and tasty formula to
increase strength and
vitality, build the blood,
and enhance the immune
system. It's best if the
herbs infuse for many
months; I often make this
in the summer and then
strain it and begin taking
it as autumn comes on,
to protect against winter
colds and flus.*

2 PARTS *PANAX* GINSENG ROOT

2 PARTS SIBERIAN GINSENG ROOT

2 PARTS ASTRAGALUS ROOT

2 PARTS CODONOPSIS ROOT

1 PART DONG QUAI ROOT

1 PART COOKED REHMANNIA ROOT

1 PART JUJUBE RED DATES

1 PART LYCII BERRIES

1 PART GRATED FRESH GINGERROOT

½ PART CINNAMON CHIPS

BRANDY

Make a tincture, following the
directions on page 14.

To use: Take 1–2
teaspoons per day, a few
days a week, during the
autumn–winter season.

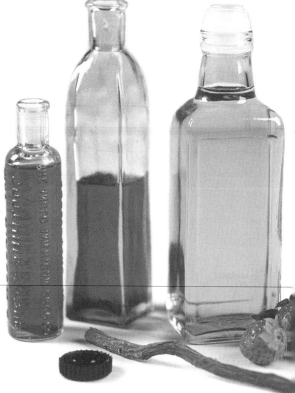

Women's Vitality Tonic

If you wish to make the 10
Treasures Vitality Tonic more
specific for women, increase
the dong quai to 2 parts
and reduce the ginsengs to
1 part each.

Min-Elix Herbal Syrup

3 PARTS ROSE HIPS

2 PARTS NETTLE LEAVES

2 PARTS WILD OATS

2 PARTS CHICKWEED, PREFERABLY FRESH

2 PARTS MALVA LEAF, PREFERABLY FRESH

1 PART YELLOW DOCK ROOT

1 PART ALFALFA LEAF

1 PART RED CLOVER BLOSSOMS

1 PART VIOLET LEAF AND FLOWER

½ PART GRATED FRESH GINGERROOT

¼ PART CINNAMON CHIPS

½ PART CHOPPED DRIED APRICOTS

½ PART CURRANTS OR RAISINS

½ PART FRESH OR DRIED CHERRIES

UNSULFURED BLACKSTRAP MOLASSES

BRANDY

RASPBERRY VINEGAR (SEE BOX)

This delicious, fruity herbal syrup is rich in easily assimilable iron and calcium. It's a great nourishing formula for children, as well as anyone feeling a little run-down or tired. It's also great as a PMS, pregnancy, postpartum, or menopausal tonic.

1. In a large pot, combine the herbs and dried fruits. Cover with 3 times as much water.

2. Bring to a boil; then reduce heat, stir well, and cover.

3. Simmer for 2 hours, stirring occasionally. Check water level as the mixture simmers; it should reduce to about half.

4. Turn off heat, and allow mixture to cool down for 2–3 hours.

5. Strain well, squeezing all liquid from the herbs. Compost herbs, and measure the volume of liquid. For every quart of liquid, add 3 cups of unsulfured blackstrap molasses, 1 cup brandy, and a few dashes of raspberry vinegar.

6. Stir well, and bottle. Store in the refrigerator; it will keep for several months.

To use: Take 1 tablespoon a few times per week over a period of several months. If you're anemic or very run-down, try 2–3 tablespoons per day, as needed.

Raspberry Vinegar

To make your own raspberry vinegar:
1. Wash and crush 2 cups of fresh raspberries.
2. Puree in a blender with 2 cups white wine vinegar or apple cider vinegar and ¼ cup honey or maple syrup.
3. Let the mixture sit overnight, then strain out seeds. Keep in the refrigerator. This vinegar can also be used in salad dressings or marinades.

Stamina City Herbal Tea

This hearty blend tastes great and is excellent for promoting general energy as well as fortifying the adrenals, blood, and metabolism. Overworked, stressed-out types, this is for you!

1 PART DANDELION ROOT	½ PART COOKED REHMANNIA ROOT
1 PART SARSAPARILLA ROOT	⅛ PART CINNAMON CHIPS
1 PART SIBERIAN GINSENG ROOT	⅛ PART LICORICE ROOT

1. In a large pot, bring 1 quart water to a boil.

2. In a bowl, mix together all ingredients. Add ½ cup of the mixture to the boiling water.

3. Reduce heat and simmer, covered, for 15 minutes.

4. Remove from heat, and steep 15 minutes. Strain.

To use: Drink 1–3 cups per day, as needed.

Sassy Root Revival

This is a strong, rooty-tooty, flavorful, hearty blend that nourishes the liver, adrenals, and blood. It's a particularly great tea for the autumn and winter months.

1 PART SARSAPARILLA ROOT	¼ PART FRESHLY GRATED GINGERROOT
1 PART SIBERIAN GINSENG ROOT	⅛ PART CINNAMON CHIPS
1 PART PANAX GINSENG ROOT	⅛ PART LICORICE ROOT
1 PART YELLOW DOCK ROOT	⅛ PART SLICED FRESH ORGANIC ORANGES*

1. In a large pot, bring 1 quart water to a boil.

2. In a bowl, mix together all ingredients except orange slices. Add ½ cup of the mixture to the boiling water.

3. Reduce heat to low and simmer, covered, for at least 1 hour.

4. Remove from heat, add oranges, and steep 10–15 minutes. Strain.

To use: Drink 1–3 cups per day, as needed.

*Leave seeds and peel intact only if using organic oranges

Neen's Amazing
Blood-Building Soup

5–7 FRESH BEETS, CHOPPED

2–3 CARROTS, CHOPPED

1 ONION, CHOPPED

SEVERAL CLOVES OF FRESH GARLIC, CHOPPED

½ CUP TOASTED BUCKWHEAT (KASHA)

½ CUP LENTILS

¼ CUP DRIED OR ½ CUP FRESH NETTLES

¼ CUP BURDOCK ROOT

1 4-INCH PIECE OF KOMBU OR WAKAME SEAWEED

1 TABLESPOON DILL WEED

1 TABLESPOON DILL SEED

1 TABLESPOON CARAWAY SEED

MISO OR TAMARI TO TASTE

FRESH LEMON JUICE OR BALSAMIC VINEGAR TO TASTE

I've been making this recipe for close to 20 years now and have seen it miraculously cure colds overnight and help people sail through stressful times. It's like a new lease on life when you're at your energy's end. Since it's easy to make, I encourage you to make a big batch and freeze some for later use.

YIELD: **2** QUARTS OF BROTH (STRAINED); ABOUT **8** SERVINGS

1. Place all ingredients except miso, lemon, and vinegar in a large soup pot. Cover with 4 quarts of water.

2. Bring to a boil and stir well. Lower heat and simmer, covered, for 2 hours.

3. Turn off heat, and allow soup to cool for 1–2 hours.

4. Strain and reserve the broth. Season the broth to taste with tamari or miso. Add a few dashes of fresh lemon juice or balsamic vinegar, as desired.

To use: Drink freely as needed to nourish and build blood, enhance energy, and ward off colds and flu. *Note:* Many people seem to want to eat this soup unstrained, rather than just drinking the broth. While most of the minerals from the vegetables are cooked into the broth itself, it's fine to consume it either way.

Hearty Miso–Shiitake Soup

This easy and delicious soup is wonderful at the turn of the seasons, when autumn is just setting in and the craving for warm nourishing soups begins. Simple to make, and oh-so-tonifying for your digestive and immune systems, this soup is a wonderful tonic for health and vitality.

YIELD: 4 CUPS; ABOUT 4 SERVINGS

3 CARROTS, CHOPPED

3 STALKS CELERY, CHOPPED

1 ONION, CHOPPED

½ CUP CHOPPED SHIITAKE MUSHROOMS

½ CUP CHOPPED OYSTER MUSHROOMS

1 TABLESPOON GRATED FRESH GINGERROOT

MELLOW WHITE OR LIGHT MISO TO TASTE (UP TO ¼ CUP)

SAKE, MARSALA, OR CREAM SHERRY TO TASTE

FRESH SCALLIONS, CHOPPED (OPTIONAL)

FRESH PARSLEY, CHOPPED (OPTIONAL)

1. In a large pot filled with 1 quart water, add the carrots, celery, onion, and mushrooms. Simmer for 15 minutes.

2. Turn off heat, and stir in ginger; miso; and sake, marsala, or cream sherry. Garnish with chopped fresh scallions and parsley, and serve. For an unusual twist, add a bit of chopped fresh rosemary and thyme to the soup just before serving. The fresh herbs add even more flavor and healthy properties.

To use: Enjoy 1–2 cups of soup for a light but nourishing meal, especially if you're feeling run-down.

Cooking with Miso

Never boil miso; doing so kills the flora that are beneficial to the digestive tract. Instead, dissolve the miso in a small amount of warm water, then add it to the soup at the end of cooking, once the heat has been turned off.

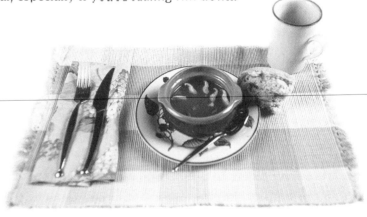

The Coffee Break

2 PARTS *PANAX* GINSENG

2 PARTS SIBERIAN GINSENG

1 PART CODONOPSIS ROOT

1 PART ROASTED DANDELION ROOT

1 PART ROASTED CHICORY ROOT

½ PART GRATED FRESH GINGERROOT

⅛ PART CINNAMON CHIPS

HONEY (OPTIONAL)

1. In a large pot, bring 1 quart water to a boil.

2. Add herbs. Simmer, covered, for 30 minutes.

3. Turn off heat, and steep another 15 minutes.

4. Strain and add a little honey, if desired.

To use: Enjoy 1–3 cups per day, as needed.

For those of you who are trying to quit the "habit" or just want a tonifying alternative, this recipe is a delicious, roasty-toasty blend with excellent tonic properties from the ginseng, codonopsis, dandelion, and chicory. This formula actually helps strengthen the adrenals, which caffeine depletes over time.

Herbal-a-Go-Go Energy Elixir

2 PARTS *PANAX* GINSENG

2 PARTS SIBERIAN GINSENG

1 PART ASTRAGALUS ROOT

1 PART CODONOPSIS ROOT

1 PART GINKGO LEAVES

1 PART NETTLE LEAVES

1 PART SLICED FRESH ORGANIC ORANGES*

½ PART GRATED FRESH GINGERROOT

¼ PART CINNAMON CHIPS

PORT WINE

BRANDY

1. Make the base by mixing together half port wine and half brandy.

2. Place all herbs in a widemouth jar. Make a tincture as instructed on page 14, using 3 times as much base as herbs.

3. After straining, sweeten lightly with maple syrup if desired; I usually add about ¼ cup maple syrup per quart of elixir.

To use: Take 1 tablespoon several times per week, as needed.

The base of this elixir is port wine and brandy, which give a deep ruby red color and nice warming qualities. This gorgeous tonic has deep blood-building and immune-enhancing properties. It can be taken any time of the year but is especially helpful in the autumn–winter season.

*Leave seeds and peel intact only if using organic oranges

Christopher Hobbs

WILLIAMS, OREGON

Christopher Hobbs, L.Ac., A.H.G., is an internationally respected fourth-generation botanist, clinical herbalist, and licensed acupuncturist. He has dedicated his life to the study of healing plants and our relationship with them. Christopher has written 20 books on health and herbal medicine, including *Herbal Remedies for Dummies, Natural Liver Therapy,* and *Foundations of Health.* He maintains a busy private practice, lectures internationally, and is developing a community healing and learning center called the Living Farmacy.

When asked about his favorite herbs, Christopher replies, "My two favorite tonics are American ginseng and ligustrum. American ginseng is a cooling and energy-enhancing North American herb that supports adrenal function and hormone production in the body while counteracting stress and chronic inflammation. *Ligustrum lucidum* berries, which are a sexual, adrenal, and hormonal tonic, also support immune function and help prevent cancer, neurasthenia, and hormonal weakness."

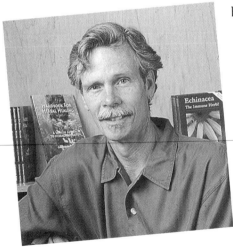

According to Christopher, tonics are herbs and foods that support body processes, provide nutrients, and offer biochemical/energetic factors that promote greater health in all the cells, tissues, and organs of the body. He recommends daily use of tonics, for three to nine months or longer for long-term conditions, but cautions that they should be discontinued for a week or 10 days during an acute infection, such as the flu or a urinary tract infection.

For more information on Christopher Hobbs and his work, visit www.allherb.com or www.christopherhobbs.com. ⊕

Wei Qi Protective
Vitality Soup

5–7 STICKS ASTRAGALUS

1 MEDIUM REISHI MUSHROOM

2–3 SMALL SHIITAKE MUSHROOMS

1/3–1/2 CUP SLIGHTLY SPROUTED BEANS, SUCH AS ADZUKI OR BLACK BEANS

1/2–1 CUP ORGANIC BARLEY

1 CUP TOTAL VEGETABLES OF CHOICE, SUCH AS CARROTS, CELERY, CABBAGE, POTATOES, CHARD, AND KALE

2–3 PIECES SEA VEGETABLES SUCH AS NORI, DULSE, OR WAKAME (OPTIONAL)

1/3 CUP FRESH OR 2 TABLESPOONS DRY GOBO (BURDOCK ROOT; OPTIONAL)

1 CUP FRESH NETTLES OR OTHER WILD EDIBLE GREENS

2–4 CLOVES GARLIC

1–2 MEDIUM ONIONS, CHOPPED

MISO OF CHOICE TO TASTE

Chris Hobbs developed this deeply tonifying soup to nourish the immune system. It can be drunk 1–2 times per week to increase resistance and stamina, or it can be consumed daily for more chronic, degenerative immune diseases. If you are very weak and run-down, you can drink the broth by itself. Make enough for a few days, and store in the refrigerator.

YIELD: ABOUT 2 QUARTS OF SOUP; 6–8 SERVINGS

1. Fill a large soup pot with 3 quarts of purified or spring water

2. Add the astragalus, reishi, shiitake, and beans and bring to a boil. Lower heat and simmer for 20 minutes.

3. Add barley, and simmer for another 20 minutes.

4. Add the vegetables, burdock, nettles, garlic, and onions and simmer until tender, about 15–20 minutes.

5. Season with miso and any favorite spices, such as ginger, celery seed, and fennel. Remove astragalus before serving; it's too woody to eat.

To use: Enjoy a hearty bowl daily, as desired. For autoimmune diseases, such as lupus, or conditions such as allergies, diabetes, and hepatitis, eat the soup and drink the broth as desired.

Donna Cerio
SANTA CRUZ, CALIFORNIA

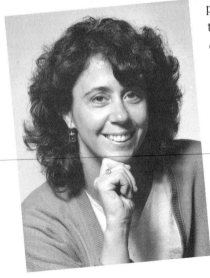

donna C. Cerio's 20 years as a health professional include alternative health care and stress management in private practice, academic settings, and the public arena. Founder and Director of the Cerio Institute, she has developed and refined a body of work that invites clients to participate in their own health care in a meaningful and effective way.

As the founding director of the Holistic Health Program at the University of California at Santa Cruz, Donna has trained and certified thousands of staff and students for 20 years. She is a certified instructor of massage, acupressure, anatomy, and physiology, as well as the author of *My Body, My Energy, My Self,* a book and cassette that begin a holistic exploration of "Who am I?" for very young children and people in recovery from early childhood trauma. She has a private practice in Santa Cruz County and delivers educational seminars and on-site services locally and across the nation.

Donna's use of herbs and foods dates back to her early childhood, when she spent countless hours in the kitchen with her mother, grandmother, and great-grandmother, absorbing their passions and talents for using foods and herbs as medicines. In her early 20s, Donna extensively studied the system of Polarity and the Eastern Medical Model. Donna has a precise and deep understanding of the role herbs and food play in building and maintaining optimal energy and health. She incorporates her knowledge into her private practice, and treats her family to natural foods — embodying her ancestors' passion for preparing fresh, wholesome meals. Donna's garden is a delight to all, sporting herbs, vegetables, and an array of colorful flowers. ⚘

Summer Cleansing
and Fortifying Salad

¼ CUP FLAXSEED OIL

¼ CUP OLIVE OIL

1 CLOVE CRUSHED GARLIC

8 GREEK OR ITALIAN OLIVES, OR 4 OF EACH, PITTED AND SLICED

3 FRESH GREEN ONIONS, CHOPPED

1 CUP BALSAMIC VINEGAR

1 TABLESPOON SWEET BASIL

1 TABLESPOON ROSEMARY

1 TABLESPOON THYME

2 SWEET PEPPERS, ONE YELLOW, ONE RED, THINLY SLICED

3 TOMATOES, SLICED

2 CARROTS, THINLY SLICED

2 HEADS OF DARK GREEN LEAFY LETTUCE,* WASHED AND BROKEN INTO BITE-SIZED PIECES

SEA SALT TO TASTE

½ CUP CHOPPED PARSLEY

½ CUP CHOPPED CHIVES

Donna says, "This is a salad that feeds the senses of smell and sight, as well as delights the taste buds. The ingredients provide the body with important vitamins and minerals, fiber, nutrition, tissue support, and disease prevention. I eat this salad 5 times per week in the summertime, and this is why all of my friends like to eat at my house!"

YIELD: 6–8 SERVINGS

1. Pour the oils into a wooden bowl, and spread the oils onto the sides and bottom of the bowl.

2. Add the garlic, olives, and green onions. Use a wooden spoon to gently spread them over the whole bowl. Repeat this process with half of the balsamic vinegar, sweet basil, rosemary, and thyme. Allow to sit at room temperature for 15 minutes.

3. Stir in the peppers, tomatoes, and carrots. Add the lettuce, toss, and allow to sit at room temperature for 5 minutes.

4. Add the remaining basil, rosemary, and thyme; some salt to taste; and the parsley. Toss well. Add more balsamic vinegar if desired.

5. Sprinkle the top with chives. Serve in festive bowls.

To use: Enjoy a bowl of salad several times per week, or as desired.

*Choose two different kinds that are in season in your area

Wild Nettle Chowder

This is one of my favorites. It's a fantastic soup, and it is easy to make if you have access to fresh nettles. Many people have a great fear of nettles, having been stung by them at some point. But nettles, once cooked, are no longer able to sting and are one of the most delicious and nutritious of all wild greens — high in protein, iron, calcium, magnesium, and vitamins A and C.

YIELD: 1 QUART OF SOUP; ABOUT **4** SERVINGS

½ TEASPOON OLIVE OIL

1 ONION, CHOPPED

3 CARROTS, CHOPPED

4 CUPS FRESH NETTLES, WASHED AND CHOPPED

MARSALA OR SHERRY TO TASTE

TAMARI TO TASTE

2 BAKED POTATOES, PEELED

FRESH OR DRIED DILL WEED AND TARRAGON TO TASTE

1. Heat the olive oil in a sauté pan over medium heat. Gently sauté the onions for 5 minutes, stirring often.

2. Add the carrots, nettles, and a few dashes of the marsala or sherry. Cover pan and steam for 5 minutes, stirring once or twice.

3. Add a dash or two of tamari, and more liquid (marsala, sherry, or water) as needed to prevent scorching.

4. Place ingredients in a blender. Add the potatoes, and puree until smooth. Add water as needed to facilitate blending.

5. Season with the dill and tarragon. Serve plain, or garnish with a dollop of yogurt or sour cream.

To use: Enjoy 1–2 cups of soup for a hearty and delicious energy boost.

Choosing Nettles

The flavor of nettles is quite pleasant, subtly nutty and unique. If you are able to collect your own fresh nettles, use the young spring tops, before the plant has gone to bloom. If you live in an area where there aren't any nettles, you can substitute another type of wild or store-bought edible greens, such as spinach, kale, chard, or bok choy.

Immune Tonics: Building Our Natural Defenses

The soups, teas, syrups, and cordials in this chapter offer a tasty array of immune-enhancing options. In the true spirit of tonifying and strengthening, these recipes are specific for building resistance to wintertime bugs. Start thinking about winter health in the early autumn, which is a great time to start making and benefiting from these recipes.

Although some of these recipes could be used as remedies for acute conditions, they are wonderful preventive formulas, meant to enhance your capacity to fight off germs. With such good-tasting and intriguing recipes at hand, staying healthy has never been more fun!

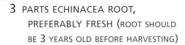

Winter Shield Protective
Echinacea–Elderberry Tincture

This is one of the most delicious tinctures imaginable, with a strong berry flavor that's hard to resist. I use this tried-and-true standby whenever there are a lot of people getting sick around me, and when I travel during the winter. It can be used at the first onset of a cold or flu, during the acute phase, and on through the tail end of the illness.

3 PARTS ECHINACEA ROOT, PREFERABLY FRESH (ROOT SHOULD BE 3 YEARS OLD BEFORE HARVESTING)

2 PARTS BLUE ELDERBERRIES, FRESH OR DRIED

2 PARTS ROSE HIPS

1 PART FRESH OR FROZEN BLACKBERRIES

1 PART FRESH OR FROZEN RASPBERRIES

1 PART GRATED FRESH GINGERROOT

1 PART SLICED FRESH ORGANIC ORANGES*

BRANDY

Make a tincture, following the directions on page 14.

To use: Take 1 teaspoon 1–5 times per day, as needed.

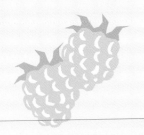

Building Up the
Natural Defenses

I usually take 1 teaspoon of Winter Shield formula per day as a preventive dose, a few days each week, in the autumn–winter season. If I travel on airplanes or it's the height of cold and flu season, I take 1 teaspoon daily for a week or two. If you're actually coming down with an acute cold or flu, you can increase the dose to 1 teaspoon about every 3–4 hours. If you're making this remedy for children, tincture it in ½ brandy and ½ vegetable glycerin; this will reduce the alcohol content to about 20 percent and will give a sweet, syrupy quality to the tincture.

*Leave peel and seeds intact only if using organic oranges

Enhancing Vitality
Herbal Soup

2 STICKS ASTRAGALUS ROOT

2 STICKS CODONOPSIS ROOT

1 SMALL WHOLE DONG QUAI ROOT, OR A FEW THIN SLICES OF THE BIGGER ROOTS

1 3-INCH PIECE OF *PANAX* GINSENG ROOT

1 CUP BARLEY OR RICE

1 3-INCH PIECE OF KOMBU OR WAKAME SEAWEED

1 ONION, CHOPPED

3 CARROTS, CHOPPED

2 STALKS CELERY, CHOPPED

2 YAMS, CHOPPED

1 ZUCCHINI, CHOPPED

2 TABLESPOONS GRATED FRESH GINGERROOT

3 TABLESPOONS DRIED, OR ½ CUP FRESH, BURDOCK ROOT

MISO OR TAMARI TO TASTE

This soup incorporates the ancient Chinese custom of simmering strengthening herbs into soup stock. When I've had soups like this, the first sip is like instant rejuvenation — the ahhh, I-feel-10-years-younger effect. The herbs used here are full of immune-enhancing properties, and this soup always comes out rich and hearty. You can add any vegetables you might have on hand; squashes and root vegetables, such as turnips and rutabagas, are nice embellishments.

YIELD: ABOUT 2 QUARTS OF SOUP; 8 SERVINGS

1. Fill a large soup pot with 3 quarts water. Add the astragalus, codonopsis, dong quai, and ginseng and simmer, covered, for 1 hour.

2. Add the rest of the ingredients except for the miso and tamari, and simmer for another 30 minutes or so. (If you like, you can add some organic chicken or soup bones at this point; it's traditional in China to make this soup with chicken.)

3. Remove from heat and season with miso or tamari. Remove the astragalus before serving. If you'd prefer to eat the codonopsis, donq quai, and ginseng along with the rest of the soup, chop them before serving.

To use: Enjoy a hearty bowl of soup 2–3 times per week in the autumn–winter season.

Making this colorful and festive elixir has become a tradition in my herb classes. This antiviral formula is loaded with fresh vitamin C and bioflavonoids, and it really helps keep you healthy during cold and flu season. It's one of the most visually pleasing and utterly fabulous-tasting cordials, and its demulcent nature is oh-so-soothing for sore throats. This elixir is appropriate for children, too.

2 PARTS FRESH LEMON BALM

2 PARTS FRESH CALENDULA BLOSSOMS

2 PARTS FRESH ROSE HIPS (DRY WILL WORK FINE, TOO)

2 PARTS FRESH, RIPE, MASHED PERSIMMON

1 PART FRESH FENNEL

1 PART SLICED FRESH ORGANIC ORANGES OR TANGERINES*

1 PART GRATED FRESH GINGERROOT

¼ PART CINNAMON CHIPS

2 PARTS FRESH ECHINACEA LEAVES AND/OR ROOTS (OPTIONAL; ENHANCES THE ANTIVIRAL ACTION)

BRANDY

Make an elixir, following the directions on page 16.

To use: Adults can enjoy 1–2 tablespoons of this delightful formula several days per week throughout the autumn–winter season. For children, use ¼–½ teaspoon several days per week throughout the autumn–winter season.

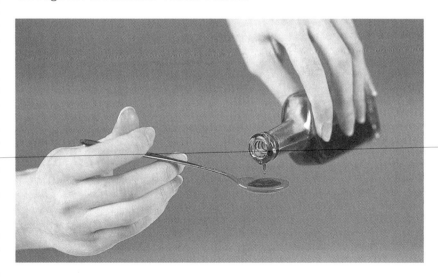

*Leave seeds and peel intact only if using organic fruit

Steamin' Mama's Lemonade

JUICE OF ONE FRESH MEDIUM
LEMON

2 CUPS BOILED WATER

1–2 TABLESPOONS HONEY OR MAPLE
SYRUP

⅛–¼ TEASPOON CAYENNE PEPPER

Stir the fresh lemon juice into the hot water. Add the honey or maple syrup and the cayenne pepper, and stir well.

To use: Drink 1–2 cups as needed at the first sign of chills, sore throat, or cough. Sip slowly, and be prepared to "feel the heat"! Can be drunk as often as needed; generally, 2–3 times per day if you're feeling sick or a few times per week as a tonic.

This is a simple warming and antiseptic drink that is both preventive and remedial for any upper respiratory congestion (coughs, colds, flu, bronchitis, and so forth). This drink requires that you keep a box of tissues nearby!

YIELD: 2 CUPS

Autumn Tonic Tea

2 STICKS ASTRAGALUS ROOT

2 STICKS CODONOPSIS ROOT

3 TABLESPOONS SARSAPARILLA ROOT

3 TABLESPOONS ROASTED DANDELION
ROOT

2 TABLESPOONS GRATED FRESH
GINGERROOT

1 TABLESPOON CINNAMON CHIPS

1 TABLESPOON LICORICE ROOT

1. Simmer all the herbs, covered, in 1 quart of boiling water for ½ hour.

2. Turn off heat, and allow to steep for another ½ hour.

3. Strain, and drink 1–2 cups per day, several days per week.

As the summer ends it's time to start thinking about nourishing herbal teas. By tonifying in the fall, I have had many healthy winters over the past 10 years — while most everyone around me suffers with long, drawn-out colds and flus. This simple tea boosts immunity; start drinking it in early November.

YIELD: 3 CUPS

Osha-Ginger Syrup

This is a delectable way to benefit from osha, a powerful, warming anti-viral herb with a bitter, aromatic, maple-type flavor. The honey base helps disguise osha's bitter flavor. This syrup is appropriate for dry, raspy coughs; sore throats; and other upper respiratory irritations. Kept in the refrigerator, the syrup will last for months. **Note:** Do not use osha during pregnancy.

YIELD: 2 CUPS

2 CUPS HONEY

¾ CUP GROUND OSHA ROOT

¾ CUP ROSE HIPS

½ CUP GRATED FRESH GINGERROOT

BRANDY (FOR AMOUNT, SEE STEP 5)

1. Pour the honey into a widemouthed quart jar. Stir in the osha, rose hips, and ginger.

2. Fashion a "double boiler" by placing the jar into a pan of gently simmering water. The level of the water in the pan should be no more than halfway up the jar. Simmer over low heat for 1–2 hours, stirring often.

3. Turn off the heat, and allow the syrup to cool for 1 hour.

4. Strain, using cheesecloth or a nylon straining bag. It's a bit messy to strain, but worth it!

5. Measure the final volume of the syrup, and add ¼ cup brandy for every cup of syrup. Store in refrigerator.

To use: Take 1 teaspoon–1 tablespoon as needed as a cough syrup or for sore throats.

Cyclone Cider Deluxe

¼ CUP GRATED FRESH GINGERROOT

¼ CUP CHOPPED ONION

¼ CUP FRESH ROSEMARY LEAVES

⅛ CUP FRESH SAGE LEAVES

⅛ CUP GRATED FRESH HORSERADISH

4 SLICES FRESH ORGANIC LEMON*

4 SLICES FRESH ORGANIC ORANGE*

4–6 FRESH PEELED GARLIC CLOVES

2–4 CAYENNE PEPPERS

APPLE CIDER VINEGAR

HONEY OR MAPLE SYRUP

This is a variation on an old favorite among herbalists, serving as both a syrup and as a very interesting addition to soups, stews, salad dressings, and marinades. Once you make it, you might find you can't live without it; it's a bold statement to any silly germs who thought they might invade you!

YIELD: APPROXIMATELY 1½ QUARTS

1. Place all herbs, fruits, and vegetables into a widemouthed jar. Cover with 2–3 times as much apple cider vinegar.

2. Place plastic wrap over jar and then secure tightly with a lid. Shake daily for 2–4 weeks. Store at room temperature out of direct heat and light.

3. Strain, squeezing all liquid possible out of the herbs.

4. Discard herbs and rebottle the vinegar. Add honey to taste, enough to make a syrupy consistency (roughly equal parts vinegar and honey).

To use: Take 1–2 tablespoons as needed, or add to soups, sauces, marinades, and dressings.

*Leave seeds and peel intact only if using organic fruits

Ray Swartley
BIG SUR, CALIFORNIA

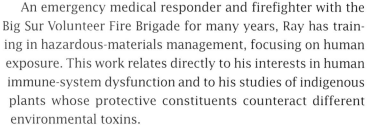

ay Swartley is a lifelong holistic-somatic massage practitioner, herbalist, gardener, and trailblazer living in Big Sur, California. He is a member of the Esalen Institute Massage and Teaching Staff and teaches workshops in massage, herbology, and experiential awareness practices at Esalen and throughout Europe. Ray looks to nature's systems and their inherent healing capacities, which support awareness, understanding, and change. He uses yoga and meditation techniques as a preparation for experiencing the healing properties of herbs and essential oils.

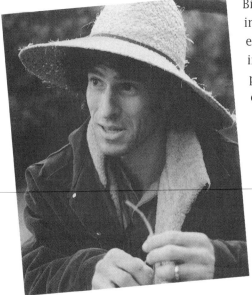

An emergency medical responder and firefighter with the Big Sur Volunteer Fire Brigade for many years, Ray has training in hazardous-materials management, focusing on human exposure. This work relates directly to his interests in human immune-system dysfunction and to his studies of indigenous plants whose protective constituents counteract different environmental toxins.

Ray says, "I work from a place of deep reverence and compassion. I have an underlying concept of what balance, harmony, and fluid grace can look and feel like. My work supports movement and breath, providing room for change and internal clearing. My practice and teaching focus on human-botanical relationships, using indigenous wild medicinal plants and essential oils to integrate mind, body, and spirit."

Big Creek Lung Formula

4 PARTS FRESH ARALIA ROOT, CHOPPED

3 PARTS GRATED FRESH GINGERROOT

3 PARTS DRIED OSHA ROOT, SHREDDED
   OR GRATED

2 PARTS FRESH FALSE SOLOMON'S SEAL
   ROOT, CHOPPED

2 PARTS FRESH FENNEL, CHOPPED

2 PARTS FRESH DOUGLAS FIR TIPS OR
   PINE NEEDLES, CHOPPED

2 PARTS FRESH OR DRIED ROSE HIPS

2 PARTS FRESH ORGANIC ORANGES,
   CHOPPED*

2 PARTS YERBA SANTA LEAVES,
   CHOPPED

2 PARTS FRESH MALVA LEAVES,
   CHOPPED

BRANDY OR EVERCLEAR, DILUTED TO 60
   PERCENT ALCOHOL CONTENT

Make a tincture as directed on page 14.

To use: As a preventive tonic during cold and flu season, take 1–2 dropperfuls per day, a few days per week. After the onset of illness, take 1–2 dropperfuls 3–5 times per day.

Every spring Ray collects fresh wild herbs and makes this spicy, warming, antiviral tincture that wards off colds, flus, and coughs. Be sure you positively identify aralia before using; it has several poisonous look-alikes. If you can't find fresh aralia and false Solomon's seal, you can substitute store-bought dried angelica root and marsh mallow root, respectively.

*Leave seeds and peel intact only if using organic oranges

Ray's Warming Winter Brew

2 PARTS FRESH LEMON BALM

2 PARTS FRESH CATNIP

2 PARTS FRESH SAGE

2 PARTS FRESH THYME

2 PARTS GRATED FRESH GINGERROOT

1 PART FRESH OR DRIED ROSE HIPS

½ PART LICORICE ROOT

Make an infusion by following the directions on page 12.

To use: Drink 1–2 cups per day as a preventive tonic or 3–4 cups per day for acute colds and flu.

The herbs in this tea are common in many gardens and are easy to grow. This is a great choice if you want to fortify yourself against winter "bugs," and it also can be used as an antiviral for acute colds and flu. It tastes good, too!

Mary Nosse
Santa Cruz, California

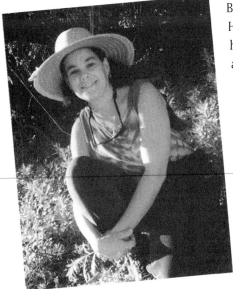

from an early age, Mary Nosse remembers wanting to know the mysteries of plants, including their names, properties, and growing seasons. In her teens she worked in health food stores and became interested in herbal cosmetics and remedies. She was often found concocting healthy cookies or fragrant facial steams, and was labeled the "mad scientist" by her father. Now, at the end of the '90s, Mary finds herself a wife, mother, and corporate assistant caught up in the world of fast food, coffee, computers, and stress. Fortunately, she has rediscovered her herbal roots and reawakened her love of the plant world.

Mary recently completed a two-year apprenticeship with Botanic Adventures, assisting me in my 10-month Deepening Herbal Perspectives course. Combining her business skills with her love of plants, Mary incorporates gardening, healthy cooking, and lots of creative product-making into her busy life. Over the course of 1999, "Proud Mary's" kitchen took on a life of its own, and now her counters and cupboards are lined with innumerable colorful homemade cordials, salves, liniments, and tinctures.

Embracing the study of herbs outdoors as well reading and doing on-line research, Mary has reclaimed her former alchemist-like interest in plants. Her favorite all-around herbs are burdock, comfrey, eucalyptus, ginger, ginseng, spearmint, and yarrow. Reports Mary, "They are simple, effective herbs that are easily grown or found in nature and have such deep and profound effects on human health." ◈

Proud Mary's "Rolling on the River" Mind-Loving Tonic

1 PART ANISESEED

1 PART ARAME SEAWEED*

1 PART ASTRAGALUS ROOT

1 PART BURDOCK ROOT

1 PART CHICKWEED, FRESH IF POSSIBLE

1 PART GINKGO LEAVES

1 PART NETTLE LEAVES

1 PART *PANAX* GINSENG ROOT

This unusual and tasty tincture benefits the mind, circulation, digestion, and immune system. It is rich in minerals and can be a nice boost in the autumn, strengthening the body and increasing vitality before winter arrives.

1. Place all ingredients in a widemouthed glass jar. Cover with 3 times as much brandy, making a tincture as instructed on page 14.

2. Once the tonic is strained, you may turn it into a cordial by lightly sweetening it with maple syrup (see directions for making cordials on page 16).

To use: Enjoy 1–2 teaspoons per day, a few days per week, in the autumn–winter season.

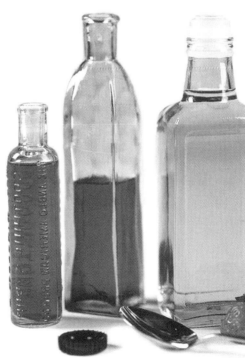

*Available in natural foods stores

Garlic–Ginger Syrup

I find this recipe extremely easy to prepare, and it makes a wonderful preventive tonic during cold and flu season. It's effective against viruses and bacteria and can be taken by the spoonful for warding off sore throats, colds, and coughs. It's so tasty that you can add a spoonful or two to salad dressings, marinades, soups, and more.

YIELD: 2½ CUPS

2 CUPS HONEY

½ CUP PEELED FRESH GARLIC CLOVES

½ CUP GRATED OR SLICED FRESH GINGERROOT

1. Gently warm the honey over very low heat for 1–2 minutes, until it's thin and runny. Do not boil the honey.

2. Place the garlic and ginger into a widemouthed jar. Pour the honey over the herbs and stir well. Secure with a lid.

3. Store in a warm, sunny place for 3 days. Stir daily.

4. Refrigerate the syrup. Use within 1–2 months.

To use: Enjoy the syrup by the spoonful. For an antiseptic hot toddy, add 1–2 tablespoons to a cup of hot water, with a bit of fresh lemon. You can eat the "pickled" garlic and ginger, too.

Syrup with a Twist

For a more adventurous twist on the Garlic–Ginger Syrup, add ½ cup apple cider vinegar and ¼ cup tamari to each cup of syrup. Experiment by adding a spoonful or two to sauces, salad dressings, soups, and marinades. Keep the syrup in the refrigerator between uses.

Brain Tonics & Memory Enhancers

Mental clarity? What's that?

Are you the academic type? Computer whiz? Creative type? Do you find you wish you had more focus, better memory, more creative juices flowing through the ol' noggin? Well, believe it or not, there are herbal tonics that work specifically to enhance memory and recharge brainpower. How about something as yummy as Smart Cookies Persimmon–Vanilla Cordial, or Herbal Brainstorm Rosemary–Raspberry Lemonade? With a little experimentation and the following recipes, you can have a really good time making and taking your tonics!

Golden Glow
Ginkgo–Gotu Kola–Siberian Ginseng Tincture

Fresh ginkgo leaves are traditionally harvested in the late summer, just as they start to turn golden yellow. It is thought that this is when the active flavones, which are largely responsible for ginkgo's tonic action, are at their peak. This formula is very simple yet powerful, and it enhances blood flow and oxygen to the brain.

1 PART GINKGO LEAVES

1 PART GOTU KOLA LEAVES

1 PART SIBERIAN GINSENG ROOT

BRANDY

Make a tincture, following the directions on page 14.

To use: Enjoy ¼–1 teaspoon per dose, 1–3 times per day, as needed.

If I Only Had a Brain Tea

When you have to study, write, or think impressive and creative thoughts, this tea will promote mental clarity. It's a nice alternative to coffee and black tea, and much more gentle and fortifying for your nervous system.

2 PARTS SIBERIAN GINSENG ROOT

1 PART GOTU KOLA LEAVES

1 PART GINKGO LEAVES

1 PART PEPPERMINT LEAVES

1. In a large pot, add the ginseng to 1 quart boiling water. Reduce heat and simmer, covered, for 20 minutes.

2. Turn off heat. Add the remaining herbs and steep for 20 minutes.

To use: Drink 2–3 cups per day.

Smart Cookies
Persimmon–Vanilla Cordial

2 PARTS GINKGO LEAVES

2 PARTS SIBERIAN GINSENG ROOT

2 PARTS ROSE HIPS

2 PARTS HAWTHORN BERRIES

1 PART FRESH, RIPE, MASHED PERSIMMON

1 PART FRESH LEMON BALM OR LEMON VERBENA

1 PART SLICED FRESH ORGANIC ORANGES OR TANGERINES*

1 PART GRATED FRESH GINGERROOT

¼ PART CINNAMON CHIPS

1 VANILLA BEAN, SLICED LENGTHWISE AND CUT INTO ¼-INCH SLIVERS

BRANDY

HONEY OR MAPLE SYRUP

Make a cordial, following directions on page 16.

To use: Enjoy 1–2 tablespoons per day, a few days per week (more, of course, if you're on a big holiday shopping spree!)

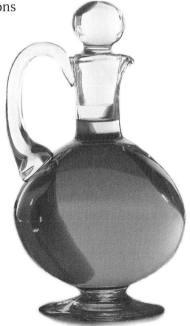

This is a delightful holiday cordial to give to your friends and family. It's colorful and delicious and has true brain- and stamina-enhancing properties. It's perfect for people who need to think clearly while they "shop till they drop" around the holidays.

*Leave seeds and peel intact only if using organic fruit

Wake-Up Call Herbal Tea

This is a nice, noncaffeinated morning tea to refresh and stimulate your mind and senses. Many of the olden European herbals refer to rosemary and sage as herbs to "comfort thy braine," increase memory, and enhance wisdom.

*Leave seeds and peel intact only if using organic fruit

2 PARTS PEPPERMINT LEAVES

2 PARTS ROSE HIPS

1 PART GINKGO LEAVES

1 PART GRATED FRESH GINGERROOT

1 PART LEMON BALM OR LEMON VERBENA

¼ PART ROSEMARY LEAVES

¼ PART SAGE LEAVES

¼ PART SLICED FRESH ORGANIC ORANGES OR TANGERINES*

⅛ PART STAR ANISE PODS OR FENNEL SEEDS

Make an infusion, following the directions on page 12.

To use: Enjoy 2–4 cups per day, hot or iced.

Green Drink Delight

This fresh-blended drink supplies lots of vital magnesium-rich chlorophyll, vitamins, and minerals. It's a great pick-me-up for any time of day or night. Green drinks are also a great way to build your blood.

YIELD: ½ CUP

*Chickweed, miner's lettuce, plantain, young dandelion leaves, young yellow dock leaves, purslane, and lamb's-quarter are good choices

¼ CUP CHOPPED FRESH EDIBLE WILD YOUNG GREEN HERBS OF CHOICE*

¼ CUP PINEAPPLE JUICE OR APPLE JUICE

¼ CUP WATER

1. Place all ingredients in blender. Blend at high speed until pureed.

2. Strain through a strainer, pressing all liquid out of herbs.

To use: Take ¼ cup at a time, 1–2 times per day. Refrigerate any leftovers and use within 24 hours.

Ginkgo–Strawberry–Peach Love Wine

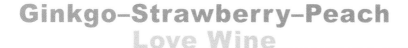

1 750-ML BOTTLE OF WHITE ZINFANDEL WINE

2 CUPS FRESH GINKGO LEAVES, OR 1 CUP DRY GINKGO LEAVES

¼ CUP FRESH STRAWBERRIES

1 RIPE PEACH, SLICED

¼–½ CUP HONEY OR MAPLE SYRUP

1. Place all ingredients except honey or maple syrup in blender. Pulse the blender on and off until ingredients are lightly blended.

2. Pour the mixture into a widemouthed jar. Secure the lid and shake well. Infuse overnight at room temperature.

3. Refrigerate the following day, and continue to infuse in the refrigerator for 1–2 weeks.

4. Strain well, squeezing all liquid possible from the mixture. Sweeten lightly with honey or maple syrup. Kept refrigerated, the wine will last for months.

To use: Consume in 3- or 4-ounce portions as a late-afternoon aperitif or drink a small wineglassful before dinner. It's also delightful to sip with meals, but be careful of how much you drink!

Well, since I've heard more than once in my life that the brain is the "largest organ of romance," I thought I might include this sublime recipe for enhancing the brain — and then let nature take its course! This is quite tasty; you may have to restrain yourself from consuming more than just a wee bit.

YIELD: 1 QUART

Supercharger
Morning Smoothie

This highly nutritious and yummy smoothie packs a wallop of protein, fresh vitamins and minerals, and extra "brain food" to get you going in the morning. It helps set you up for an active, productive day, so whip this up and blast off to work or play.

YIELD: ABOUT 12 OUNCES;
1 LARGE SERVING

1 CUP FRESH-SQUEEZED ORANGE OR TANGERINE JUICE

¼ CUP FROZEN BANANA CHUNKS

¼ CUP SLICED FRESH OR FROZEN PEACHES

2 TABLESPOONS SOY–VANILLA PROTEIN POWDER (OR FLAVOR OF YOUR CHOICE)

1 TABLESPOON SPIRULINA POWDER*

1 TEASPOON LECITHIN GRANULES*

1 DROPPERFUL OF GINKGO TINCTURE OR GLYCERITE (GLYCERIN TINCTURE)*

1 DROPPERFUL OF SIBERIAN GINSENG TINCTURE OR GLYCERITE (GLYCERIN TINCTURE)*

Blend all ingredients in a blender until smooth.

To use: Sip and enjoy!

Why Add Tinctures
to Smoothies?

The idea of adding a tincture to a smoothie may be novel to some of you. The amount of alcohol in the 2 dropperfuls of tincture is so minimal that it shouldn't affect the taste. A nice alternative is a glycerite, or glycerin tincture, which is alcohol-free. If the tinctures mentioned in the recipe above are not readily available or you don't like the idea of adding them, simply leave them out.

*Available at most health food stores

Herbal Brainstorm Rosemary–Raspberry Lemonade

1 QUART WATER

¼ CUP FRESH OR ⅛ CUP DRY ROSEMARY LEAVES

3 MEDIUM-SIZED LEMONS

¼–½ CUP HONEY OR MAPLE SYRUP

1 CUP FRESH OR FROZEN RASPBERRIES

ICE CUBES

EDIBLE FLOWERS FOR GARNISH

1. Make a rosemary infusion, following the directions on page 12. Stir, cover, and allow to steep for 15–20 minutes.

2. Strain out the rosemary leaves, and add the fresh lemon and honey or maple syrup. Stir well and transfer to a festive glass bowl.

3. Add the raspberries and ice cubes, and garnish with a few sprinkles of edible flowers.

To use: Enjoy by the glassful as a special tonic at parties, luncheons, or other gatherings.

This beautiful, refreshing drink is a fusion of herbs, flowers, and good old-fashioned lemonade. It can be served iced or warm, and it really gives a nice lift to the brain. A great party drink, this treat can be sipped on a hot summer day when you have to think brilliantly.

YIELD: ABOUT 1½ QUARTS

Scrumptious Edible Flowers

Some of my favorite edible flowers include:

* Bachelor's buttons (cornflowers)
* Basil blossoms
* Borage
* Calendula
* Dianthus (sweet William)
* Johnny-jump-ups and pansies
* Lavender
* Nasturtiums
* Rose geraniums
* Rose petals
* Rosemary blossoms
* Sage blossoms
* Thyme blossoms

Rosemary Gladstar
EAST BARRE, VERMONT

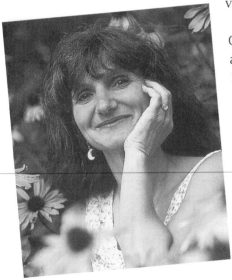

osemary's grandmother, Mary Egitkanoff, had the earliest influence on this renowned herbalist. In the early 1900s, Mary survived the near genocide of the Armenian people. She felt that her strong belief in God and her extensive knowledge of plants saved her life during this time, and she passed her knowledge on to her grandchildren.

Rosemary's herbal apprenticeship continued into her early 20s, when she lived and backpacked extensively throughout the Pacific Northwest. She credits the launch of her herbal career to a "true-life adventure and dream come true": In 1971 she successfully navigated a long stretch of the California Coastal Trail on horseback, surviving almost exclusively on wild foods, roots, herbs, and berries.

In 1972, Rosemary opened her first herbal store, Rosemary's Garden, in Sebastopol, California. An educator, businesswoman, and medical consultant working with doctors and hospitals, Rosemary is also the author of several herb books and has created and managed many successful product lines. But first and foremost, Rosemary considers herself an earth-based community herbalist who also promotes plant restoration.

To Rosemary, herbal tonics offer a bracing and uplifting experience. She says, "Tonics are those herbs that build, strengthen, and enhance life-function. I find it amazing that the word 'tonic,' the most important term in herbal therapy, is not even recognized by allopathic medicine."

It's no surprise that Rosemary's favorite herbs include nettle, burdock, dandelion, and Siberian ginseng, all known for their nourishing, adaptogenic, and vitality-enhancing properties. She advises, "Life should be a tonic. Plants, sunshine, fresh-flowing water, good air, and refreshing activity are all part of the great tonic formula for a healthy life."

Rosemary's warm and gracious nature has blessed all those who know her. Almost 30 years since she offered her first class, Rosemary continues to inspire students worldwide through her writings and teachings.

Long-Life Elixir

¼ PART SAW PALMETTO BERRIES

1 PART ASTRAGALUS ROOT

2 PARTS SASSAFRAS ROOT BARK

2 PARTS FO-TI-TIENG

2 PARTS DAMIANA LEAF

2 PARTS GINGERROOT

2 PARTS LICORICE ROOT

1 PART CHINESE STAR ANISE PODS

2 PANAX GINSENG ROOTS PER QUART OF TINCTURE

BLACK CHERRY CONCENTRATE*

1. Make a tincture by following the directions on page 14. Steep for 6–8 weeks; the longer, the better.

2. When the tincture is done steeping, strain and discard the herbs. To each cup of liquid add ¼ cup black cherry concentrate. Though it's tasty, do not add more than ¼ cup of concentrate per 1 cup of tincture, as this may cause fermentation.

3. Shake well to mix, and rebottle. If desired, add the ginseng roots back into the rebottled elixir.

To use: Take about ⅛ cup 2–3 times per week for a few months at a time.

Rosemary came up with this recipe's name by chance. The first time she made the elixir, she stored it in an antique glass bottle that had engraved upon it "The Tree of Life" and the words "Long Life." The name seemed fitting and has stuck. This tonic builds strength and vitality, and though it can be enjoyed by both sexes, it is predominately a yang, masculine-type tonic.

*Available at health food stores; do not use fruit juice

7-Herb Long-Life Soup

This wonderful recipe from Rosemary can incorporate any number of tonic and/or adaptogenic herbs. A highly nourishing and restorative blend, 7-Herb Long-Life Soup is an excellent broth to serve to someone recovering from illness. Use fresh herbs if possible, and use other seasonings and chopped vegetables if desired. This soup may also be made with organic chicken.

YIELD: 2 QUARTS; 8 SERVINGS

2 ONIONS

2–3 CLOVES OF GARLIC

1 TABLESPOON OLIVE OIL

3 QUARTS WATER

2 OUNCES FO-TI (HO SHOU WU)

2 OUNCES ASTRAGALUS

2 OUNCES LYCII BERRIES

¼–1 OUNCE GINSENG ROOT (CAN BE ANY VARIETY)

2–4 FRESH DANDELION ROOTS, SLICED INTO THIN PIECES (OR 2 OUNCES DRIED)

4–6 FRESH BURDOCK ROOTS, SLICED INTO THIN PIECES (OR 4 OUNCES DRIED)

1 TABLESPOON FRESH GINGERROOT

4 LARGE SHIITAKE MUSHROOMS (FRESH OR DRIED), CHOPPED

MISO TO TASTE

1. Sauté the onions and garlic in olive oil until tender and golden.

2. Heat the water. When boiling, add all ingredients. Reduce heat to low and allow to simmer for several hours. Stir occasionally.

3. When the roots are tender, turn off heat and strain out the herbs. (I often leave the herbs in, especially if they are fresh.) Add miso to taste (do not boil the miso). Enjoy a bowl as desired.

Brain-Tonic Tincture

Rosemary's tonic is specific for enhancing memory. If you're picking your own fresh ginkgo, pick the leaves in late summer; this is when their flavonoid content is highest and they are most potent.

2 PARTS GOTU KOLA

2 PARTS GINKGO LEAF

1 PART PEPPERMINT LEAF

¼ PART SAGE

¼ PART ROSEMARY

Make a tincture, following the directions on page 14.

To use: Take ¼–1 teaspoon, diluted in a little warm water or juice, daily for 1–2 months.

Healthy Heart & Circulatory Tonics

So often, people associate a "healthy" diet with deprivation. What's good for the heart can't possibly be luscious or fun to consume, right? Well, this chapter offers several nourishing "heart-healthy" recipes that are as tasty as can be.

In these modern times of ever increasing stress and busy-ness, it's relaxing and therapeutic to simply slow down and make tonics, enjoy them, and share them with friends. Strengthening your connection to the plants, to the earth, and to the loved ones with whom you share these special formulas . . . well, that's good medicine for the heart. In the spirit and tradition of sharing good food and festivities, here are a few of my all-time favorite tonics.

Hawthorn–Ginkgo
Heart–Brain Tonic

I've been making this tonic for years, using hawthorn, rose hips, and ginkgo, which are flavonoid-rich, to nourish and strengthen the heart, circulatory system, and brain. In Europe younger family members pick fresh hawthorn berries in the autumn, then make a delicious syrup to present at Christmas to the elders in the family.

2 PARTS HAWTHORN BERRIES

2 PARTS HAWTHORN LEAVES AND
FLOWERS (AVAILABLE AT HERB STORES
AND THROUGH MAIL ORDER)

2 PARTS ROSE HIPS

1 PART GINKGO LEAVES

1 PART SLICED FRESH ORGANIC ORANGES
OR TANGERINES (LEAVE SEEDS AND PEEL
INTACT IF USING ORGANIC FRUIT)

1 PART RIPE PLUM, PITTED AND CHOPPED

1 PART FRESH OR FROZEN RASPBERRIES

BRANDY

Make a cordial by following the directions on page 16.

To use: Take 1–2 tablespoons per day, several days per week.

Heart's Ease Tea

This blend is excellent for relaxing and nourishing the heart and cardiovascular system. The hawthorn, ginkgo, and motherwort are cardiotonic, while the linden, wild oats, and motherwort are also relaxing and antispasmodic.

3 PARTS HAWTHORN LEAVES AND
FLOWERS

2 PARTS HAWTHORN BERRIES

2 PARTS GINKGO LEAVES

2 PARTS MOTHERWORT LEAVES

2 PARTS WILD OATS

2 PARTS VIOLET LEAVES AND FLOWERS

1 PART LINDEN BLOSSOMS

Make an infusion by following the directions on page 12.

To use: Enjoy 2–3 cups per day, a few days per week.

Herbal Better Butters

Well, it's not a tea or cordial, and you may wonder why I'm introducing something with the dread word "butter" in the title! Blending butter, oil, and herbs, Better Butters are culinary delights that are easy to make, extraordinary to cook with, and much more heart healthy than margarine or pure butter; the saturated fat and cholesterol are cut in half, and heart-healthy omega-3 fatty acids are introduced.

Better butters are also easy to spread. Just think: no more waiting for cold, hard butter to soften! The variations are endless, but here are a few of my favorites.

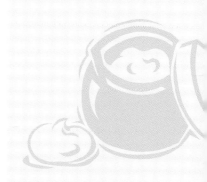

Garlic–Herb Better Butter

½ CUP (1 STICK) SOFTENED BUTTER

½ CUP OLIVE OIL

2–3 TABLESPOONS MINCED FRESH GARLIC

2 TABLESPOONS PAPRIKA

2–4 TABLESPOONS CHOPPED FRESH (OR 2 TABLESPOONS DRIED) BASIL, ROSEMARY, TARRAGON, OR DILL

2 TABLESPOONS SUN-DRIED TOMATO BITS

1. In a bowl, mix all ingredients well with a wooden spoon.

2. Cover, and store in refrigerator (it will last 1–2 weeks) or freezer (freeze in small batches; lasts indefinitely). If frozen, defrost as needed. If dried herbs are used, the butter will last for several weeks when refrigerated.

This particular better butter is fantastic for garlic bread; when melted over baked potatoes, steamed vegetables, popcorn; or when used as a base to sauté with. It's so flavorful, you'll find you don't need to use as much in cooking, which will also benefit your heart.

YIELD: 1⅓ CUPS

Orange–Honey Better Butter

This better butter is great on cornbread, pancakes, morning pastries, and so forth. It's so good, you may have to make it more often than you'd imagine!

YIELD: 1⅓ CUPS

½ CUP (**1** STICK) SOFTENED BUTTER

½ CUP ORGANIC SAFFLOWER OR FLAX OIL

⅓ CUP HONEY

3 TABLESPOONS GRATED FRESH ORANGE OR TANGERINE RIND

1. In a bowl, mix all ingredients well with a wooden spoon.

2. Cover, and store in the refrigerator; it will last for 1–2 weeks. If frozen in small batches, it will last indefinitely. Defrost as needed.

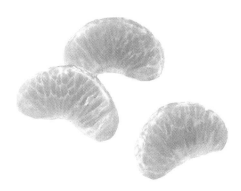

Pineapple–Rose Honey Butter

You may have to keep this one under lock and key. I've seen people of all ages ooh and aah over it, even eating it straight. It does seem to have some kind of magical effect and an ambrosia-like fusion of flavors.

Follow the recipe above for Orange–Honey Better Butter. Add to it 2 tablespoons crushed, drained pineapple, ¼ cup minced fresh rose petals (or 2 tablespoons dried and crumbled), and 1 teaspoon vanilla extract. Stir all ingredients well, and store in a covered container in the refrigerator. It will last 1–2 weeks if refrigerated, or indefinitely if frozen. If frozen, defrost the butter as needed.

Balsamic Blast

½ CUP EXTRA-VIRGIN OLIVE OIL

⅛ CUP SHERRY—MAPLE BALSAMIC
    VINEGAR (SEE BOX)

4–6 CRUSHED FRESH GARLIC CLOVES

1 TABLESPOON GRATED FRESH
    PARMESAN OR ROMANO CHEESE

1 TABLESPOON FRESH CALENDULA
    PETALS

1 TEASPOON FRESH BASIL LEAVES

1 TEASPOON FRESH ROSEMARY LEAVES

1 TEASPOON FRESH LEMON THYME
    OR REGULAR THYME LEAVES

1 TEASPOON DRY-ROASTED WHOLE
    CORIANDER SEEDS (SEE BOX)

½ TEASPOON DRY-ROASTED WHOLE
    BLACK PEPPERCORNS (SEE BOX)

½ TEASPOON GRATED FRESH
    ORANGE RIND

¼ TEASPOON CRUSHED RED CHILI
    FLAKES

This is a colorful, savory, heart-healthy alternative to butter. Various creative versions of this are easy to make, once you get the basic concept down. In California, many Italian and "California Cuisine" restaurants serve some kind of basic rendition of balsamic vinegar and olive-oil dipping sauces, but I've not seen any as good as this!

YIELD: ABOUT ¾ CUP

1. Pour the olive oil into a shallow bowl or onto a couple of big plates. Drizzle the vinegar over the olive oil.

2. Sprinkle the rest of the ingredients on. Enjoy as a dipping sauce for warm, crusty sourdough or French bread or as an unusual salad dressing.

Secret Ingredients

Years ago, I tried a very expensive 25-year-old oak-aged balsamic vinegar. It was so good I had to figure out how to make regular balsamic vinegar taste like that. I mixed together 1 cup balsamic vinegar, ⅓ cup cream sherry, and ¼ cup maple syrup, and voilà! I had my own rendition.

To dry-roast coriander and black peppercorns, heat a heavy-bottomed skillet over low—medium heat for 1 minute. Add the coriander seeds and black peppercorns and stir for a couple of minutes, until the coriander turns golden brown.

Hawthorn–Rose Hips Conserve

This recipe is so incredibly delicious and good for you (even fat-free!) that you may wonder how you ever lived without it. Unfortunately, it doesn't have a long shelf life, so eat it up once you make it! Great food for the heart and soul.

YIELD: 2½ CUPS

½ CUP HAWTHORN BERRIES, FRESH IF POSSIBLE

1 CUP ROSE HIPS (IF USING DRY, PURCHASE THE SEEDLESS "CUT AND SIFTED" ROSE HIPS)

¾ CUP HONEY

2 TABLESPOONS FRESH LEMON JUICE

1 TABLESPOON VANILLA EXTRACT

1 TEASPOON CINNAMON POWDER

1. Boil 2 cups water. Add the hawthorn berries and turn down heat. Cover and simmer for 1 hour, stirring often.

2. Turn off heat, cover, and allow to steep for 1 more hour.

3. Strain, reserving the liquid. Discard berries.

4. Reheat liquid to just under boiling, and pour over the rose hips in a bowl. Cover and steep for ½ hour to soften and rehydrate the rose hips.

5. Place about ½ of the liquid (including rose hips) in a blender, then add the honey, lemon juice, vanilla extract, and cinnamon. Blend on low speed, adding more liquid as necessary to facilitate blending. The texture should be thick and puddinglike.

6. Strain through a large strainer to remove any stray seeds. This conserve is thick and gooey, so keep scraping it off the bottom of the strainer as it comes through.

To use: Try a spoonful a day as a nourishing heart and vitality tonic. Spread on pancakes, waffles, oatmeal, muffins, and other foods. It also makes a really nice topping for fruit salad, or you can mix it with yogurt or applesauce. Vitamin C–rich and soothing, this also makes a delicious "spoonful of medicine" for children or adults with sore throats, colds, or coughs. Cover and refrigerate leftovers and use within a week.

Happy-Heart Tea

2 PARTS HAWTHORN LEAVES AND FLOWERS

2 PARTS HAWTHORN BERRIES

1 PART ROSE HIPS

1 PART LINDEN BLOSSOMS

½ PART LEMON VERBENA LEAVES

½ PART MOTHERWORT LEAVES

¼ PART ORGANIC ORANGE PEEL

Make an infusion, following the directions on page 12.

To use: Enjoy 2–3 cups per day, a few days per week.

This recipe is a pleasant-tasting, gently relaxing formula that tones and fortifies the heart and nerves. The hawthorn and rose hips are flavonoid-rich and nourishing to the heart and cardiovascular system. Motherwort is glycoside rich and tones the heart and relaxes the nerves.

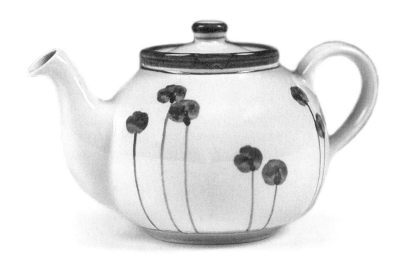

Ruselle Rubine and Raqib Lynn, L.Ac.
SANTA CRUZ, CALIFORNIA

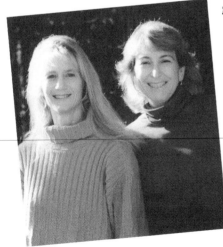

uselle Rubine has had a thriving professional massage practice in Santa Cruz since 1988. She incorporates herbal and nutritional therapies to promote relaxation, rejuvenation, and rebalancing in her clients.

Ruselle grew up playing in the open fields of Orange County, California. As a young child she loved making forts and would collect pods, flowers, seeds, and grasses for pretend food and medicine, and for beautification. In 1992, she completed the first class of the American School of Herbalism in Santa Cruz. She studied for 2½ years with Christopher Hobbs and Michael Tierra, learning Chinese as well as western herbalism. Now her kitchen counter is covered with jars of herbs in alcohol or oil, and herbs are hanging everywhere to dry. Ruselle can often be found in her huge garden, enjoying the energies of the fresh plants.

Ruselle was president of the Santa Cruz Herb Coalition from its inception. But mostly, she just loves plants! One of her favorite herbs is licorice root because of its sweetness and harmonizing qualities. "It is the sugar that helps the medicine go down in the herbal world, and it's such a great tonic."

Raqib Lynn also maintains a private practice in Santa Cruz. As an acupuncturist and herbalist, she has been in full-time practice since 1991. Raqib teaches Chinese herbology and Chinese medical theory throughout the United States and abroad, in locations such as Ireland and Israel. She is a faculty member of the American School of Herbalism in Santa Cruz and is well known for her enthusiastic, informative, and organized lecture style.

Working, studying, and playing with herbs since the mid-1980s, Raqib has myriad favorite herbs. At the present time, she names lycii berries as one of her favorites, for their fortifying and nourishing properties for the blood, liver, and eyes. In Raqib's life and work, herbs play a fundamental role in optimal daily health. ♧

Hawthorn Syrup

4 CUPS HAWTHORN BERRIES

4 CUPS WATER

4 CUPS HONEY

JUICE OF ½ LEMON

CINNAMON TO TASTE

1. Collect hawthorn berries when ripe and dark red (usually in October). Rinse and remove stems and seeds (like pits).

2. In a large pot, combine the berries and water. Bring to a boil, then lower heat.

3. Simmer for about 6 hours, stirring occasionally, until the liquid is reduced to almost half the original amount. Berries will be soft and can be mashed at this point to make mixture thick and soupy.

4. After mashing the berries, stir well. Measure the volume of liquid; you should have approximately 1 quart.

5. Add honey, and bring just to boiling. Be careful: The mixture can foam up and make a big mess! If necessary, lower heat.

6. Turn off heat and add the lemon juice. Add cinnamon or other flavorings, about ½ teaspoon for each cup of syrup. Get creative!

7. Pour into mason jars; allow to cool. Add clean lids and refrigerate.

To use: Use fresh or chilled as needed for healthy treats.

Ruselle's simple yet tasty syrup can be used on hot cereal, pancakes, waffles, and more. It's fabulous with these comfort foods because it seems to help the heavy carbohydrates be digested more easily — and it also nourishes the heart! It will last at least a year refrigerated (unopened), or it can be "canned." It makes a great gift! Ruselle makes enough to last a year (the amounts listed).

YIELD: 2 QUARTS

Dong Quai Chicken Soup

Raqib created this rich, hearty, and delicious blood tonic and blood builder. This is a terrific recipe for those who have never worked with raw Chinese herbs; it's a great way to demystify the entire process of cooking Chinese herbs. The soup is good for depletion of any kind, with symptoms such as tiredness, lethargy, pre- or postmenstrual fatigue, or lack of motivation.

YIELD: 1½ QUARTS; 6 SERVINGS

3 SLICES DONG QUAI

3 PIECES CODONOPSIS (DANG SHEN)

5 PIECES WILD YAM (DIOSCOREA)

1–2 OUNCES JOB'S TEARS (COIX BARLEY)

1.5 OUNCES LYCII BERRIES

1 SMALL ORGANIC CHICKEN, CUT INTO PIECES

1 ONION, SLICED

1 CARROT, SLICED

5–10 LARGE KALE OR COLLARD LEAVES (CUT OFF STEMS)

TAMARI, SOY SAUCE, OR SEA SALT TO TASTE

1. Put the rinsed herbs in a porcelain, earthen, or Pyrex pot.

2. Add 10 cups water. Heat to a boil, and then reduce and simmer for 2 hours.

3. Add chicken. Cook for 45 minutes or until fully cooked. Add vegetables, plus the tamari, soy sauce, or sea salt to taste, and cook until tender (about 15–20 minutes).

To use: The dong quai will dissolve in cooking. The lycii and Job's tears are edible and delicious. The codonopsis and dioscorea will swell up considerably; although they are edible, a little nibble is probably all you will want to try. Serve with white or basmati rice, and provide a small bowl for bones and inedible herb remains. If you don't use the whole pot of soup in one meal, try cooking some fresh greens every time you serve it. This will make your soup more attractive, more delicious, and more healthful.

Men's Tonics: Strength & Vitality Enhancers

It's no secret that men and women alike are burning the candle at both ends these days. Jobs are stressful, life is demanding, freeways are more crowded, and the cost of living is skyrocketing. No wonder fatigue is such a common complaint. What would it be like to have more energy? How about a little extra vitality? Is there life beyond caffeine? Read on to find out.

The following recipes are each one-of-a-kind. They're awesome. They are unlike anything you can buy in the store, so resign yourself: You are about to become a real man who makes herbal tonics!

The recipes in this chapter are invigorating for the male glandular system, and they contain traditional western and Chinese herbs to nourish and build vitality, protect and strengthen the heart, increase overall stamina, and tone the reproductive system.

Beast Juice Energy Tonic

I've been making this for years, and most of my women friends fight over it or steal it from their boyfriends. It's a superb, deep-acting tonic for building up energy, vitality, and stamina. Move over Geritol and Viagra — this fun-to-take, iron-rich tonic builds the blood, strengthens the immune system, and adds pizzazz. It takes a while to make; I usually start it in the summer and let it steep until autumn. This is the king of all tonics — great for men and women!

3 PARTS *PANAX* GINSENG

3 PARTS SIBERIAN GINSENG

2 PARTS ASTRAGALUS ROOT

2 PARTS CODONOPSIS ROOT

2 PARTS YELLOW DOCK ROOT

2 PARTS NETTLE LEAVES

2 PARTS SARSAPARILLA ROOT

2 PARTS WILD OATS

2 PARTS ROSE HIPS

2 PARTS HAWTHORN BERRIES

1 PART LYCII BERRIES

1 PART RED JUJUBE DATES

1 PART FO-TI-TIENG ROOT

1 PART DRIED APRICOTS

1 PART RAISINS OR CURRANTS

1 PART GRATED FRESH GINGERROOT

BRANDY

APPLE CIDER VINEGAR

UNSULFURED BLACKSTRAP MOLASSES

MAPLE SYRUP

1. Place all herbs and dried fruits in a widemouthed 1-gallon jar. Cover with 3 times as much of a mixture of half brandy and half apple cider vinegar.

2. Cover top of jar with plastic wrap to prevent rusting, secure lid, and shake well.

3. Continue shaking daily for first month, then put jar in a dark cupboard and allow to sit for 2 months; shake every few days.

4. Strain, squeezing all liquid possible out of the herbs. Compost herbs, and measure volume of liquid. For every quart of liquid, add 2 cups molasses and 1 cup maple syrup. Stir well.

To use: Take 1–2 tablespoons per day, a few days per week. If very tired or run-down, take 1–2 tablespoons a few days in a row, then ease back to a few days each week. Women can also take it on an occasional basis throughout the autumn–winter season or when in need of a deep energy boost. Keep refrigerated; it will last indefinitely.

Ginseng Swing Herbal Tea

2 PARTS SIBERIAN GINSENG ROOT

1 PART DANDELION ROOT

1 PART HAWTHORN BERRIES

1 PART SARSAPARILLA ROOT

⅛ PART CINNAMON CHIPS

¹⁄₁₀ PART LICORICE ROOT

¹⁄₁₀ PART ORANGE PEEL

Make a decoction, following the instructions on page 13.

To use: Enjoy ½–1 cup per day, a few days per week.

Here's a great tonic for overall energy, stamina, and mental clarity. The hawthorn nourishes the heart; the dandelion tones the liver and digestive system; and the Siberian ginseng, sarsaparilla, and licorice nourish the adrenals and male glandular system.

Tarzan's Total Tonic

2 PARTS *PANAX* GINSENG ROOT

2 PARTS SIBERIAN GINSENG ROOT

2 PARTS SARSAPARILLA ROOT

2 PARTS MEDJOOL DATES, MASHED

1 PART FO-TI-TIENG ROOT

1 PART SAW PALMETTO BERRIES

1 PART NETTLE LEAVES

1 PART WILD OATS

1 PART HAWTHORN LEAVES AND FLOWERS

1 PART HAWTHORN BERRIES

1 PART SLICED FRESH ORGANIC ORANGES*

⅛ PART CINNAMON CHIPS

⅛ PART LICORICE ROOT

Make a cordial, following the directions on page 16.

To use: Take 1–2 teaspoons per day, a few days per week.

This tonic is easy to make and tastes pretty good (considering that it's full of some less-than-delicate-tasting herbs). It benefits the male reproductive organs and glandular system, and builds up the male hormonal system and energy level.

*Leave seeds and peel intact only if using organic oranges

"In the Mood" Damiana-Orange-Chocolate Cordial

Well, the title says a lot about this particular cordial. Damiana was once known as Turnera aphrodisiaca *and has enjoyed a long and colorful history as an "herb of love." There are many variations on damiana cordials, but here's one of my favorites.*

YIELD: 3 CUPS

1 OUNCE DAMIANA LEAVES

1 VANILLA BEAN, SLICED LENGTHWISE

¼ CUP SLICED FRESH ORANGE RIND

2 CUPS BRANDY

1 CUP HONEY OR MAPLE SYRUP

¼ CUP CHOCOLATE SYRUP

1 TABLESPOON VANILLA EXTRACT

1 TABLESPOON DISTILLED ORANGE BLOSSOM WATER*

1. Place the damiana, vanilla bean, and orange rind in a wide-mouthed jar.

2. Cover with brandy, cover jar, and shake well every day for 2 weeks. Store at room temperature and out of direct light and heat.

3. Add the rest of the ingredients and steep for 2 more weeks, shaking daily.

4. Strain, squeezing all liquid possible from the herbs. Save the vanilla bean but discard the rest of the herbs. Rebottle cordial and add the vanilla bean back in. Let sit in a dark place for 1 more month.

To use: Sip in small amounts as a delicious love treat (for men or women) to help set the mood and enhance the senses. Sharing out of a 1-ounce port glass is nice.

*Available at health food and herb stores

Summer Superman
Energy Shake

2 CUPS FRESH-SQUEEZED ORANGE OR
  TANGERINE JUICE

1 CUP PLAIN YOGURT OR PEACH-
  FLAVORED YOGURT

½ CUP CRUSHED ICE

2 TABLESPOONS NUTRITIONAL YEAST*

2 TABLESPOONS MAPLE SYRUP

Blend all ingredients at high speed
in blender.

To use: Sip and enjoy!

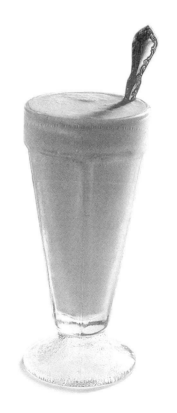

*Sometimes, something
makes a lasting impres-
sion on you. I had this
simple smoothie in March
of 1976, the day I moved
to Santa Cruz and started
at UCSC. Minutes after
drinking it, I found
myself happily sprinting
across campus, full of
vigor and energy. It's so
easy to make, you can
whip it together in a
couple of minutes and
then enjoy the benefits
for hours.*

YIELD: 3½ CUPS

Healthy Options

To the Summer Superman Energy
Shake you can add any of the following for extra pizzazz (all are
readily available in health food and
herb stores):

✳ 1 dropperful Siberian ginseng
  extract

✳ 1 small vial of *Panax* ginseng
  extract

✳ 1 small vial of royal jelly

*Available in health food
stores; this is *not* baking yeast

James Green

FORESTVILLE, CALIFORNIA

James Green is the owner and director of the California School of Herbal Studies in Forestville, California. He is the founder of Simpler's Botanical Company, which distributes tinctures, salves, and essential oils nationwide. Since 1969, James has enjoyed communing with plants and teaching about their health-promoting beauty. He is the author of the popular books *The Male Herbal* and *The Herbal-MedicineMaker's Handbook*.

Currently, James is developing a user-friendly western constitutional model of health, which helps people recognize and esteem their unique individual differences and simultaneously cherish the similarities of all human beings. In an atmosphere of appreciating oneself and one another, James inspires people to focus on health and well-being rather than on disease. He believes the plants should be embraced as uplifting allies.

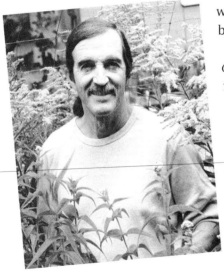

James cites stinging nettle, St.-John's-wort, and wild oat as three of his favorite tonic herbs. Nettle is appreciated for its wonderful versatility as a wild food and nourishing medicine. As a herbal-medicine maker, James reveres St.-John's-wort for the transformative alchemy of its dynamic color changes and its uplifting energetics. Wild oat is "the perfect herb for nourishing my overindulgent nervous system," says James with a twinkle in his eye. According to James, tonics are vital "because they best nourish and support who we are. As allies, we can experience a mutually nourishing plant-person appreciation. I feel that plants adore us as much as we adore them."

James's Temperament Tonic #1

1 PART DAMIANA LEAVES

1 PART ST.-JOHN'S-WORT FLOWERS

1 PART MUGWORT LEAVES

1 PART NETTLE SEED (YOU'LL PROBABLY HAVE TO HARVEST THIS YOURSELF)

1 PART ROSEMARY LEAVES

Make an infusion, following the directions on page 12, or make a tincture by following the directions on page 14.

To use: Drink 1–3 cups of tea per day, a few days a week. Or take 1–3 droppersful of tincture per day, a few days a week.

This recipe from James uplifts and stimulates the endomorphic–monarch–kapha component, which produces patterns of depression and apathy. Useful for "stagnant" individuals who tend to get depressed, withdrawn, and lethargic in stressful situations, this formula helps "brighten the chi," decongest the liver, and lift the spirits.

James's Temperament Tonic #2

1 PART SKULLCAP

1 PART GOTU KOLA

1 PART VERVAIN

1 PART PASSION FLOWER

Make an infusion, following the directions on page 12, or make a tincture by following the directions on page 14.

To use: Drink 1–3 cups of tea per day, a few days a week. Or take 1–3 droppersful of tincture per day, a few days a week.

This tonic mellows and cools the mesomorphic–warrior–pita component, which produces patterns of irritability and anger. Useful for the "excess" individual who gets easily annoyed and develops a short temper in stressful situations. This formula is also useful for hyperactive nervousness.

James's Temperament Tonic #3

1 PART AMERICAN GINSENG

1 PART WILD OAT

1 PART LAVENDER

This tonic nourishes and invigorates the ectomorphic–seer–vatta component, which produces patterns of anxiety and exhaustion. Useful for the "deficient" individual who easily becomes overburdened and fatigued when facing difficult situations, this formula helps balance, tone, and nourish the nervous system.

Make an infusion, following the directions on page 12, or make a tincture by following the directions on page 14.

To use: Drink 1–3 cups of tea per day, a few days a week. Or take 1–3 droppersful of tincture per day, a few days a week.

Choosing Your Temperament Tonic

Each of these recipes can be prepared and taken as a tea or tincture. Each Temperament Tonic formula helps to balance the effects of a predominant component in one's individual constitutional nature.

Women's Herbal Allies: Special Tonics for Life's Different Phases

Women throughout the ages have been deeply involved in the healing aspects of plant magic and medicine. Whatever phase of life a woman may be in, herbal tonics offer specific and helpful support for the female system. From building up the blood to balancing the hormones to nourishing the bones to easing the moodiness of PMS, tonic allies work in gentle and profound ways.

The following recipes are fun to make and offer a wealth of health-enhancing and vitality-boosting qualities for women of all ages.

Power Surge Female Tonic

This is the female counterpart to Beast Juice Energy Tonic (see recipe on page 64). There are many similarities between the two tonics; I invented the recipes simultaneously and intended them to fulfill certain roles. Power Surge is high in iron and calcium and has deep blood-building, energy-enhancing, and hormone-balancing effects. It's a great PMS tonic and also works well during all phases of menopause.

3 PARTS DONG QUAI ROOT

2 PARTS COOKED REHMANNIA ROOT

2 PARTS ASTRAGALUS ROOT

2 PARTS CODONOPSIS ROOT

2 PARTS NETTLE LEAVES

2 PARTS YELLOW DOCK ROOT

2 PARTS WILD OATS

2 PARTS ROSE HIPS

2 PARTS HAWTHORN BERRIES

1 PART CHINESE WHITE PEONY ROOT

1 PART CHINESE WILD YAM ROOT

1 PART JUJUBE CHINESE RED DATES

1 PART LYCII BERRIES

1 PART DRIED APRICOTS

1 PART CURRANTS OR RAISINS

1 PART GRATED FRESH GINGERROOT

½ PART CINNAMON CHIPS

BRANDY

APPLE CIDER VINEGAR

UNSULFURED BLACKSTRAP MOLASSES

BLACK CHERRY CONCENTRATE*

MAPLE SYRUP

1. Place all herbs and dried fruits in a widemouthed 1-gallon jar. Cover with 3 times as much of a mixture of half brandy and half apple cider vinegar.

2. Cover top of jar with plastic wrap (to prevent rusting of the lid), secure lid, and shake well.

3. Shake daily for 1 month, and then put jar in a dark cupboard. Allow to sit for 2 more months; shake every few days.

4. Strain, squeezing all liquid possible out of the herbs. Compost herbs, and measure volume of liquid. For every quart of liquid, add 2 cups unsulfured blackstrap molasses, 1 cup black cherry concentrate, and ½ cup maple syrup. Stir well. Keep refrigerated; it will last indefinitely.

To use: Take 1–2 tablespoons per day, a few days per week. If very tired or run-down, take 1–2 tablespoons for a few days in a row, then ease back to a few days each week.

*Available at health food stores; do not use fruit juice

Sweet Sesame–Flax
Sprinkle

½ CUP ORGANIC SESAME SEEDS

½ CUP ORGANIC FLAXSEEDS

2 TABLESPOONS BROWN SUGAR

1 TEASPOON GROUND CARDAMOM
OR CINNAMON

1. Grind the sesame seeds and flaxseeds into a fine powder, using a coffee or herb grinder.

2. Place ground seeds in a clean glass jar, and stir in the rest of the ingredients.

3. Cover jar tightly and store in freezer. (The powder won't freeze, but this keeps it nice and cold and prevents oxidation of the valuable oils in the flaxseeds and sesame seeds.)

To use: Take 2–3 tablespoons per day, as often as you like.

This recipe was created by Mindy Green, a renowned herbalist from Colorado. A delicious condiment that is high in protein and calcium, it is wonderful sprinkled on fruit salad, yogurt, or cereal, and it makes a great addition to smoothies. The essential fatty acids in flax help balance prostaglandins in the body and support the health of the endocrine and cardiovascular systems. You'll also benefit from the fiber and lignans in flax, which are known cancer preventives.

YIELD: 1 CUP

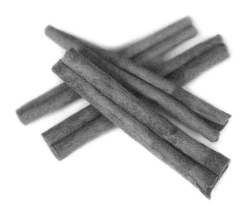

Strong Bones Cordial

This is a calcium-iron-magnesium–rich cordial that is nourishing to women of all ages and is especially important to take in the 40s and beyond. Vinegar, because of its acidity, makes an excellent base to pull calcium out of the herbs (ever hear of the old tradition of soaking eggshells in vinegar?). Unsulfured blackstrap molasses also has a fair amount of calcium and iron, making this an all-around winning formula.

3 PARTS CHICKWEED (FRESH IF POSSIBLE)

3 PARTS HORSETAIL

3 PARTS NETTLES

3 PARTS WILD OATS

3 PARTS PLANTAIN LEAVES

3 PARTS ROSE HIPS

2 PARTS FRESH MALVA (MALVA ROTUDIFOLIA OR M. NEGLECTA) LEAVES AND STEMS*

2 PARTS YELLOW DOCK ROOT

2 PARTS RED CLOVER BLOSSOMS

1 PART RASPBERRIES, FRESH OR FROZEN

1 PART CHERRIES, FRESH OR DRIED

1 PART DANDELION LEAVES

1 PART SLICED FRESH ORGANIC ORANGES OR TANGERINES**

APPLE CIDER VINEGAR

UNSULFURED BLACKSTRAP MOLASSES

1. Place all herbs and fruit into a widemouthed jar. Cover with twice as much apple cider vinegar.

2. Cover top of jar with plastic wrap (to prevent rusting of the lid), and secure lid. Shake daily for 2–4 weeks.

3. Strain well, squeezing all liquid possible out of the herbs. Compost herbs and rebottle the cordial.

4. Sweeten the cordial with 2–3 cups unsulfured blackstrap molasses per quart of cordial.

To use: Take 2–3 tablespoons per day. You can also mix the dose into ½ cup hot water for a yummy, calcium-rich, alcohol-free "toddy."

*If not available, substitute marsh mallow root

**Leave seeds and peel intact only if using organic fruit

Crybaby PMS Elixir

2 PARTS SKULLCAP LEAVES

2 PARTS WILD OATS

1 PART ST.-JOHN'S-WORT FLOWERS

1 PART LEMON VERBENA LEAVES

1 PART PASSIONFLOWER LEAVES

1 PART STRAWBERRIES, FRESH OR FROZEN

1 PART SLICED FRESH ORGANIC ORANGES OR TANGERINES*

BRANDY

Make a cordial, following the directions on page 16.

To use: Take 2–3 droppersful, as needed. If you tend to get moody during PMS, try taking 2–3 droppersful for a few days prior to menstruation each month.

Those of the female persuasion know that sometimes hormonally induced personality changes occur at the most inopportune moments. I, being a great believer in a good cry, offer this calming and centering formula for when it's not quite the right moment to let it fly.

*Leave seeds and peel intact only if using organic fruit

Nurturing Prenatal Tea

1 PART NETTLE LEAVES

1 PART RED RASPBERRY LEAVES

1 PART ROSE HIPS

1 PART SPEARMINT LEAVES

1 PART PARTRIDGEBERRY LEAVES

1 PART WILD OATS

Make an infusion, following the directions on page 12.

To use: Enjoy 2 cups per day, several days per week, before and throughout pregnancy.

This tea is mineral-rich and is excellent for strengthening and preparing the uterus for childbirth. The herbs in this recipe are classic pregnancy tonic herbs; drink the tea before and during pregnancy to help nourish the nerves, bones, and uterus.

Amanda McQuade Crawford

OJAI, CALIFORNIA

amanda McQuade Crawford, MNIMH, is a medical herbalist practicing in Ojai, California, serving the Los Angeles and Santa Barbara communities. Amanda is an internationally recognized speaker on integrated medicine and botanicals. She frequently lectures physicians at hospitals and medical schools, sharing her knowledge of traditional herb use and modern plant research. Amanda has studied and taught about natural therapies for several years in the United States and abroad.

After receiving her bachelor's degree in medieval history from Vassar, Amanda received her diploma in phytotherapy from Britain's School of Herbal Medicine. Since 1986 she has been a member of Britain's National Institute of Medical Herbalists. A founding member of the American Herbalists Guild, she has served twice on its board of directors. She is on the review committee overseeing monographs for the American Herbal Pharmacopoeia, and she serves on several professional advisory boards.

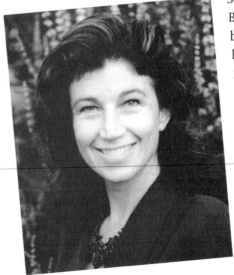

Amanda publishes articles on medical herbalism for professional journals and popular health magazines and is the author of *The Herbal Menopause Book* and *Herbal Remedies for Women.* She is the founder of the National College of Phytotherapy in New Mexico, which offers a bachelor of science program in herbal medicine. Currently, Amanda balances private practice with research for her Ph.D. in herbal medicine. ☙

Amanda's Bone-Building Tonic Tea

3 PARTS WILD OATS

2 PARTS HORSETAIL (STALKS)

2 PARTS DANDELION LEAVES

2 PARTS DANDELION ROOT

2 PARTS NETTLE LEAVES

2 PARTS CHICKWEED PLANT (WHOLE PLANT)

1 PART YELLOW DOCK ROOT

Combine all herbs, then make an infusion by steeping 1 ounce mixture in 1 quart boiling water. Steep, covered, for 20 minutes.

To use: Enjoy 2–4 cups per day.

This is Amanda's overall strengthener for the bones, nerves, skin, and hair. It is a calcium-rich tea appropriate for women during PMS or menopause and is also great for men or women as a general nourishing herbal tonic.

Amanda's Herbal Iron Elixir

4 PARTS DRIED, UNSULFURED APRICOTS, CHOPPED FINE

2 PARTS DANDELION LEAVES

2 PARTS DANDELION ROOT

2 PARTS NETTLE LEAVES

2 PARTS YELLOW DOCK ROOT

1 PART DRIED RAISINS OR CURRANTS

1 PART LICORICE ROOT

1 PART ORANGE PEEL

1 PART GRATED FRESH GINGERROOT

1. Mix all ingredients. Place 1 cup of mixture in a bowl or jar, and pour 1 quart boiling water over all. Cover and steep for 20 minutes.

2. Strain, pressing all liquid from the mixture. When cool, squeeze out liquid with a cheesecloth.

3. While it's still warm, add ¼ to ½ cup blackstrap molasses to every pint of elixir. Refrigerate, and use within 6 months.

To use: Take 1–3 tablespoons per day.

Amanda's elixir is wonderful for building up the body's iron reserves. It can be taken daily as an enriching tonic by anyone who is anemic or run-down. If you are anemic, you can take this formula for anywhere from 1 week to 3 months and then use it occasionally as needed.

Toasted Nori
Sesame Sprinkle

This is a special recipe that I made up years ago and have shared with hundreds of students in classes ever since. It is a must-have in my kitchen and is especially good on avocado sandwiches. This delicious condiment is rich in vitamin A, vitamin C, calcium, iron, protein, and minerals. It's especially appropriate for women during PMS, pregnancy, or any of the phases of menopause.

YIELD: 1 CUP

½ CUP ORGANIC SESAME SEEDS

4 SHEETS NORI SEAWEED

½ CUP NETTLE LEAVES

¼ CUP PAPRIKA

½ TEASPOON SALT

1. In a cast-iron pan over medium heat, dry-roast the sesame seeds for 1–2 minutes, stirring constantly, until golden brown.

2. Toast the nori sheets, one at a time, by waving quickly through a low flame on a gas stove. (If you have an electric stove, lightly drag each sheet of nori over the burner, using a low setting.) The nori will turn green as it toasts. When cool (this takes only a moment), crumble the toasted nori into little pieces by hand. Place in coffee grinder and pulse the grinder on and off until nori is in little flakes, about ¼ inch x ¼ inch.

3. Grind nettles into a fine powder, using coffee grinder.

4. Combine all ingredients, stir well, add salt to taste (mixture is quite flavorful; go light on salt).

5. Store in an airtight jar. Refrigeration isn't necessary.

To use: Enjoy as a condiment on salads and sandwiches, over rice and veggies, in omelettes and tofu scrambles, and more.

Digestive Tonics

Many herbalists feel that the digestive tract is central to the rest of our health. The concept of "bitters" and "carminatives" may be new to many; these are two main categories of digestive herbs. Bitters — including gentian, dandelion, angelica, Oregon grape, and mugwort — stimulate digestive juices, enzymes, and bile flow, and they help your body digest food more efficiently. Bitters also help the nutrients from your food be absorbed more efficiently. Carminatives are aromatic herbs — such as mint, cinnamon, cardamom, ginger, anise, and fennel — that stimulate digestion and also help soothe upset tummies and dispel unwanted gas. Bitters and carminatives work well together and are often combined for their flavor-balancing and synergistic action. The following recipes include some absolutely delicious teas, and some stronger bitter tonics, too. Many people (including me) find that they grow to love their bitter formulas, even crave them, and that the bitters start to taste pretty good over time!

Post-Potluck 911

What happens when four carminatives get together? They have a rollicking good time making sense out of all those weird food combinations you just ingested at that potluck dinner! This is a simple yet powerful blend to ease those post-potluck tummy woes, and it tastes good, too.

1 PART ANISE SEEDS

1 PART FENNEL (FRESH LEAVES, STALKS, FLOWERS, SEEDS, OR DRIED SEEDS)

1 PART GRATED FRESH GINGERROOT

1 PART SPEARMINT LEAVES

1. Add the anise seed, fennel, and gingerroot to boiling water, reduce heat, and simmer for 5 minutes in a covered pot.

2. Turn off heat, and add the spearmint. Steep, covered, for 15 minutes.

3. Strain, and sweeten lightly if desired.

To use: Enjoy 1–2 cups after dinner or as needed to assist digestion.

Ginger–Chamomile Delight

This tasty tea is simple and quite delicious. It's great for digestion, as both chamomile and ginger are tried-and-true carminatives, and it will help relieve stomach and/or uterine cramps. The chamomile and warm milky ginger are quite relaxing, making this a nice tea to drink before bedtime.

1 PART CHAMOMILE FLOWERS

1 PART GRATED FRESH GINGERROOT

¼ CUP COW'S, SOY, RICE, OR ALMOND MILK

HONEY OR MAPLE SYRUP TO TASTE

1. Place the herbs in a pot, and cover with boiling water.

2. Stir well, cover, and steep 15–20 minutes.

3. Strain, add the milk of your choice, and sweeten to taste.

To use: Sip slowly and enjoy as needed, preferably after dinner or before bedtime.

Ginger–Licorice Digestive Tea

1 PART GRATED FRESH GINGERROOT

1 PART PEPPERMINT LEAVES

1 PART LEMON VERBENA LEAVES

⅛ PART LICORICE ROOT

Make an infusion, following the directions on page 12.

To use: Enjoy 1–2 cups with or after meals.

This likable, flavorful blend is a great digestive tea. It also doubles as a remedy for sore throats, hoarseness, and coughs. Great hot or iced, it may win over a few skeptics.

Bahamas Bitters Digestive Tincture

1 PART FRESH MUGWORT LEAVES

1 PART FRESH FENNEL LEAVES AND STALKS

1 PART FRESH LEMON BALM

1 PART GRATED FRESH GINGERROOT

1 PART SLICED FRESH ORGANIC ORANGES OR TANGERINES*

BRANDY

Make a tincture, following the directions on page 14.

To use: Take 1 teaspoon 1–3 times per day, before or after meals, as needed.

This formula proved itself indispensable when I went to the Bahamas in 1998. I had just finished making this formula in Santa Cruz, and I threw a bottle into my pack as I headed for the islands. The food there was greasy and heavily processed and left much to be desired. For 3 weeks I took this tincture almost every day. My little bottle of Bahamas Bitters saved my digestive tract!

*Leave seeds and peel intact only if using organic fruit

Finding Fresh Mugwort and Lemon Balm

Both mugwort and lemon balm are usually poor quality when purchased in dried form; try and find them fresh. Both grow in the wild, and lemon balm is also easy to cultivate. If you can't get hold of them fresh, substitute gentian root for the mugwort and lemon verbena for the lemon balm.

Daniel J. Gagnon, Medical Herbalist

SANTA FE, NEW MEXICO

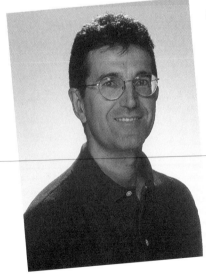

an accomplished speaker and educator, Daniel has a passion for herbs. He has been a practicing herbalist since 1976, and his goal is to educate the American public and the medical profession on the practical applications of herbal medicine. Canadian-born, Daniel relocated to Santa Fe, New Mexico, in 1979 and purchased the retail herb shop Herbs, Etc. in 1982. Herbs, Etc. is the largest and most complete herb store in the Southwest, and it manufactures a line of 132 single and formula herbal extracts that are available to natural foods stores worldwide.

Daniel is also the president of the Botanical Research and Education Institute, which publishes material on herbal therapeutics. He has authored two books and numerous articles for health and medical publications.

A few of Daniel's favorite and most essential herbs are echinacea, because it's the "quintessential herb" for stimulating the immune system and fighting off colds and flu; garlic, osha root, and yarrow for their diverse and powerful antiviral and antibiotic actions; and passionflower for its relaxing and mellowing effect.

Daniel says, "Herbal tonics are as essential to health care as exercise is. . . . Herbal tonics are like push-ups: The more you do them, the stronger your body becomes. So the key with herbal tonics is: Do them on a regular basis." Daniel's main wish is that people get well and that they know that alternatives are available. "It's important that we get back to basics, and that people learn about self-care." ☖

Daniel's Digestive Tonic

3 OUNCES CHAMOMILE FLOWERS

2 OUNCES CATNIP LEAVES

½ OUNCE FENNEL SEEDS

½ OUNCE GENTIAN ROOT

½ OUNCE ANGELICA ROOT

1. Grind and mix all ingredients.

2. Using 1 ounce of the mixture per pint of hot water, steep 20 minutes.

3. Strain, and refrigerate the liquid.

To use: Serve warm. Take 1 ounce 2–3 times a day before meals.

This tea reduces inflammation of the stomach and intestines, gets rid of gas, stops cramping, increases assimilation of foods, and sweetens the breath.

YIELD: 1 PINT

Essential Energy Builder

3 OUNCES REISHI MUSHROOMS

2 OUNCES SHIITAKE MUSHROOMS

2 OUNCES MAITAKE MUSHROOMS

1½ OUNCES ASTRAGALUS ROOT

1½ OUNCES SCHISANDRA BERRIES

1 OUNCE SIBERIAN GINSENG

½ OUNCE GINGERROOT

1. Grind and mix all ingredients.

2. Using 1 ounce of mixture per pint of water, simmer 30 minutes.

3. Strain, and refrigerate the liquid.

To use: Serve warm. Take 1 ounce of the liquid twice a day for 3 months.

This special recipe from Daniel strengthens the immune system, aids in the production of immunoglobulins, and strengthens internal organs. These herbs aid in the prevention of cancer and help to minimize the side effects of radiation and chemotherapy.

YIELD: 1½ CUPS

Suzanne Elliot

EL GRANDA, CALIFORNIA

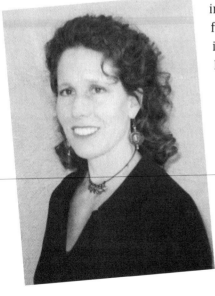

a t an early age, Suzanne Elliot acquired an enthusiasm for creating luscious meals in the kitchen with her Sicilian mom. Not long afterward, Suzanne was entrusted with preparing the family meals, which were often described as "interesting" because of her ample use of oregano.

Suzanne's interest in herbs was first sparked in 1976, while she was working in a plant nursery. She was given her first herb book during this time, and thus began her creative and enthusiastic exploration of the herbal world. "I am compelled by herbs," she says. "They constantly speak to me." To this day, her life and career are pleasantly enmeshed with the colorful and diverse world of plants.

A passion for teaching led Suzanne to offer ongoing herbal classes in Half Moon Bay, California. Utilizing plants from the wild, as well as from her beloved herb garden, Suzanne employs a hands-on approach in her teaching. She is also the owner and formulator of Woodsorrel Handmade Herbal Body and Bath Products, and runs a thriving Shiatsu therapy practice.

I met Suzanne 8 years ago at the American Herbalists Guild conference in Santa Cruz, California. We instantly recognized an alchemist's streak in each other. We sat down and started sharing herbal recipes, and haven't stopped since. Two peas from the same pod, Suzanne and I both love to concoct and consume wild and delicious herbal drinks, soups, elixirs, and more. If only we had time to cook together more often!

On the topic of herbal tonics Suzanne remarks, "Tonics are important because they help nourish and support the body and are safe for long-term use." ⊕

Garden of Eden Elixir

1 CUP DRIED FIGS, CUT IN PIECES

1 HANDFUL FRAGRANT ROSE PETALS
   (USE TWO HANDFULS IF FRESH)

3 STAR ANISE PODS

½ CINNAMON STICK, BROKEN
   INTO PIECES

½ VANILLA BEAN, SLIT LENGTHWISE
   AND CUT INTO PIECES

Make an elixir, following the directions on page 16.

To use: Slowly sip ⅛–¼ cup per serving.

This is a delectable drink to savor during the full moon or other festive occasions. Suzanne's special tonic is best sipped in small quantities, out of a decorative glass, and in the presence of good company.

YIELD: APPROXIMATELY 2 CUPS

Suzanne's Herbal Bitters

3 PARTS GENTIAN ROOT

1 PART DANDELION ROOT

½ PART YELLOW DOCK ROOT

½ PART GINGERROOT

¼ PART ORANGE PEEL

¼ PART FENNEL SEED

¼ PART CARDAMOM SEED

¼ PART LICORICE ROOT

BRANDY

VODKA

1. Place herbs in a clean jar. Fill jar with half brandy and half vodka; allow 2–3 inches of brandy–vodka covering over the herbs.

2. Seal with lid. Store at room temperature out of direct light and heat. Shake daily for 2–3 weeks.

3. Strain through cheesecloth. Compost herbs. Store the tincture in an amber bottle; it will last for several years if stored properly.

To use: Pour ½ teaspoon of the tincture in a mug, and cover with ½ cup boiling water. Add a slice of lemon. Sip in the morning, and before or after meals.

"Bitters" refer to herbs with a bitter taste that stimulate and aid the digestive process. Bitters start working, via the taste buds, as soon as you take them. Suzanne says, "It's important to challenge your taste buds, because through taste the whole digestive system is affected." This formula is tonifying for the digestive tract and is helpful for constipation, slow digestion, stomach upset, and gas.

After-Dinner
Digestive Delight

My recipe is simple but very effective for helping digestion. It's a lovely deep green, fragrant brew, and it really does ease an overly full or upset tummy. Use the herbs fresh if possible; they're easy to grow, and they make such a great fresh cup of tea!

1 PART FRESH FENNEL (LEAVES, FLOWERS, SEEDS, AND/OR STALKS)

1 PART FRESH SPEARMINT LEAVES

Make an infusion, following the directions on page 12.

To use: Enjoy 1–2 cups with or after meals.

Belly-Blast
Digestive Tincture

This strong formula for sluggish digestion is one of my all-time favorites. The bitter herbs help stimulate digestive enzymes. Great to take 15 minutes before or about 30 minutes after a big meal; it's also nice to take when traveling, when mealtimes and foods may be different than usual.

*Leave seeds and peel intact only if using organic fruit

1 PART GENTIAN ROOT

1 PART OREGON GRAPE ROOT

1 PART DANDELION ROOT

1 PART BURDOCK ROOT

1 PART YELLOW DOCK ROOT

1 PART FENNEL (FRESH IF POSSIBLE)

½ PART GRATED FRESH GINGERROOT

½ PART SLICED FRESH ORGANIC ORANGES*

⅛ PART CARDAMOM PODS

1/10 PART CINNAMON CHIPS

Make a tincture, following the directions on page 14.

To use: Take ½–1 teaspoon 1–3 times per day, as needed. You may also dilute the dose in ⅛ cup water, tea, or juice.

Herbal Detox: Balanced Formulas for Cleansing

So, you want to give up coffee or sugar for a while? Or maybe you simply want to try a modified healthy diet for a few days or a week? The following recipes are effective for short- or long-term cleansing and are very useful if you are trying to give up anything addictive — including cigarettes, caffeine, and alcohol.

Cleansing herbs assist the body by stimulating normal channels of elimination: the liver, kidneys, and bowels. Most cleansing herbs will help clear toxins and excess waste products via enzymatic pathways in the liver, and may increase the kidneys' ability to filter liquid waste. Some cleansing herbs also have mild to moderate laxative action, which helps clear the bowels and counter constipation. The recipes in this chapter are also nourishing and balancing and benefit the liver and digestive tract.

6-Root Revival Herbal Tea

This is one of my favorite recipes; it's a great liver/digestive tonic and works well to cleanse and tone the liver, blood, and digestive system. The tea can also be used to help clear skin problems and boost sluggish digestion. It's appropriate for people who are coming off caffeine, drugs, or alcohol.

1 PART OREGON GRAPE ROOT	1 PART YELLOW DOCK ROOT
1 PART BURDOCK ROOT	1 PART SARSAPARILLA ROOT
1 PART DANDELION ROOT	1 PART ECHINACEA ROOT

Make a decoction, following the directions on page 13.

To use: Enjoy 1–3 cups per day, as needed.

6-Root Revival Tincture

The above recipe also makes a great tincture, which some people may prefer. Simply place all the roots in a widemouthed jar, cover with 3 times as much brandy, and proceed as instructed on page 14.

Raging Moods Calming Nervine Tea

During detox, moods and emotions can sometimes run amok. A balanced detox plan involves supporting the physical and psychological aspects of change, so here's a soothing blend to assist in the process.

2 PARTS WILD OATS	1 PART SKULLCAP LEAVES
1 PART RED CLOVER BLOSSOMS	½ PART SPEARMINT LEAVES
1 PART LEMON VERBENA LEAVES	⅛ PART LAVENDER BLOSSOMS

Make an infusion, following the directions on page 12.

To use: Enjoy 2–4 cups per day, as needed.

Seeds of Delight
Intestinal Cleanser

2 CUPS WATER

3 TABLESPOONS AGAR-AGAR FLAKES
OR 1 TEASPOON AGAR-AGAR
POWDER*

1 QUART BLACK CHERRY JUICE

3 TABLESPOONS CHIA SEEDS*

3 TABLESPOONS FLAXSEEDS

3 TABLESPOONS PSYLLIUM SEEDS

½ CUP DRIED CURRANTS, RAISINS,
OR CHOPPED FIGS

1. Bring the water to a boil. Lower heat and stir in agar-agar.

2. Bring the agar-agar to a boil, stirring constantly. Adjust heat so it doesn't boil over. Boil for 2 minutes, stirring constantly.

3. Stir the juice, seeds, dried fruit, and boiled agar-agar together in a bowl. Cover and refrigerate; the mixture will gel as it cools. The tea will last several days if stored in the refrigerator.

To use: Try 1 cupful per morning, for several days in a row. Drink plenty of water throughout the day, and try not to eat heavy, greasy, or cheesy foods. (Sorry, no ice cream or pepperoni pizza!)

This recipe works best if combined with a diet based on fresh fruits, vegetables, and grains, without any heavy dairy products. Make sure you drink lots of water to assist in the cleansing of your digestive tract. Use black cherry juice, not concentrate.

YIELD: 6 CUPS

*Available in herb and natural foods stores

Burdock–Nettle
Nourishing Tea

1 PART BURDOCK ROOT

1 PART CHAMOMILE FLOWERS

1 PART NETTLE LEAVES

1 PART RED CLOVER BLOSSOMS

⅛ PART CINNAMON CHIPS

Make an infusion, following the directions on page 12.

To use: Enjoy 1–3 cups per day.

This formula is grounding, mineral-rich, and cleansing. Burdock, red clover, and nettles all nourish and cleanse the blood and lymphatic system.

Triple Dandy Detox Tea

To many people, dandelion is a pesky weed worthy of poisoning with toxic herbicides, but dandelion is a welcome sight on my lawn. This simple recipe is a gentle yet powerful detox tea for your liver and blood. It is also nutritive, tasty, and mineral-rich.

YIELD: 1 QUART

¼ CUP RAW DANDELION ROOT

¼ CUP ROASTED DANDELION ROOT

¼ CUP DANDELION LEAVES

1. Place the herbs in a clean 1-quart canning jar. Pour boiling water over the herbs, filling jar to the top. Stir well.

2. Cover jar and infuse for several hours or overnight.

3. Strain; compost the herbs.

To use: Take 2–4 cups per day a few days per week as a mild tonic, or take 2–4 cups daily for a few days or weeks for a more powerful cleansing tonic.

3-in-1 Rebuilding Energy Tea

This is an excellent tonic for rebuilding the adrenals and nervous system in the post-detox phase. The Siberian ginseng and rehmannia nourish the kidneys and adrenal glands, the hawthorn nourishes the heart, and the wild oats feed the nervous system.

2 PARTS SIBERIAN GINSENG ROOT

1 PART HAWTHORN BERRIES

1 PART WILD OATS

1 PART COOKED REHMANNIA ROOT

1 PART NETTLE LEAVES

1. Simmer the Siberian ginseng, hawthorn, wild oats, and rehmannia in 1 quart boiling water for 30 minutes, covered.

2. Add the nettles and steep, covered, for another 30 minutes.

3. Strain; compost the herbs.

To use: Take 2–4 cups daily, several days per week, over several weeks or months.

David Howard
BIG SUR, CALIFORNIA

growing up along the coast of California, David Howard developed a strong connection to the natural world and a great love for its verdant beauty and abundant diversity. After dabbling in several unfulfilling careers, David returned to his life's work with plants. Through David's 20 years of studying and teaching healing modalities and practices, plants have continued to inspire him in a soulful and intuitive way.

"For the root of wellness to flourish and whole healing to occur, we must reestablish the integrity of our relationship with the natural world," says David. Seeking a place of natural beauty and vitality in which to work firsthand with this concept of healing, David was serendipitously led to the Growing Edge Retreat Center in Big Sur, California.

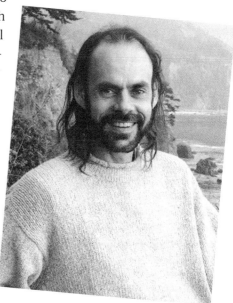

A nonprofit center, the Growing Edge emphasizes bioregional sustainability, traditional healing practices, and proactive health care. Currently, David codirects the Growing Edge, runs the botanical studies programs, and assists individuals in developing healing lifestyle programs. ⊕

Liven Up Your Liver Juice!
(a.k.a. Digestive Jubilation Brew)

This is a powerful blend. As a source of high-energy health support, herbal juices are often overlooked or unavailable unless you make them yourself. Formulated as a liver cleanser, deconges-tant, and nourisher, this brew is tops (and roots!). Enliven your system with a splash of liquid herbal essence in conjunction with a spring cleansing regimen, or any time stagnation raises its sluggish head.

YIELD: 8 OUNCES

2–3 CARROTS

1–2 STALKS OF CELERY

1 SMALL BEET

1 HANDFUL FRESH DANDELION LEAVES

1 1–2-INCH SECTION OF FRESH GINGERROOT

SEVERAL SPRIGS EACH OF FRESH PARSLEY, FENNEL, AND CILANTRO

¼ TEASPOON FRESH OR POWDERED TURMERIC

1. Juice all ingredients together except turmeric powder (if using fresh turmeric, combine with other herbs in the juicer). If using a centrifuge-type juicer, run herbs and greens through first to get the most juice from them. If you don't have a juicer, see the box below for an alternative juicing method.

2. Add turmeric if using powder. Stir well and enjoy immediately.

To use: Drink only 4–6 ounces at a time, sip slowly, and dilute with water if you find the taste or effect too strong.

Liver Juice Options

If you don't own a juicer, try dicing all fresh vegetables and herbs. Place them in a blender, add 2 cups water, and blend on high speed for 2 minutes. Strain out the pulp; refrigerate juice.

If you wish, add small amounts of any of the following fresh ingredients to your Liver Juice:

* Burdock root
* Chickweed (whole plant)
* Mugwort or yarrow tips
* Nettle tips
* Thistle greens
* Young plantain leaves

Soothing Blends for Stress and Insomnia

What's there to worry about? Stress? Perhaps it's the job that you have, or the one that you want, or maybe it's the direction your relationship is or isn't going, or maybe it's the stock market. Is it your actual life, or your worries about your life, that stresses you out the most? How about the ever increasing cost of living, finding housing, and hectic traffic? Or maybe it's world politics or environmental issues that trouble you?

Whatever the reasons, stress and worries are a very real part of our lives — and this is an area where herbs can really help. The following recipes are full of nervine tonic herbs, to soothe, nourish, and tone the nervous system. Many of the recipes are also antispasmodic and can be useful for physical tension and pain.

Spaz-Away Tincture

1 PART FRESH VALERIAN ROOT

1 PART CHAMOMILE FLOWERS

1 PART FRESH ST.-JOHN'S-WORT
   FLOWERS

1 PART WILD OATS

½ PART SLICED FRESH ORGANIC
   ORANGES OR TANGERINES*

BRANDY

Make a tincture, following the directions on page 14.

To use: Take ½–1 teaspoon 1–3 times per day, as needed.

I was having a perfectly normal day about six years ago, walking and shopping around downtown Santa Cruz. Out of nowhere, the name "Spaz-Away" popped into my head. I knew I had to make a formula to fit the name. This remedy is soothing, calming, and antispasmodic for the nerves and the body. Go ahead, try some for those bothersome "spaz attacks," whether the origin is physical, emotional, or altogether inexplicable!

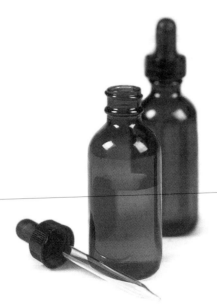

Alternatives to Fresh Herbs

In my opinion, fresh valerian root and fresh St.-John's-wort work much better than the commercially dried herbs. If the fresh herbs aren't available, you can opt to buy fresh tinctures of these two, make your own chamomile–wild oats tincture, and then mix equal amounts of the tinctures together.

*Leave seeds and peel intact
only if using organic fruit

The Cousin-of-Spaz-Away Tea

1 PART CATNIP LEAVES

1 PART CHAMOMILE FLOWERS

½ PART HOPS FLOWERS

½ PART RED CLOVER BLOSSOMS

½ PART SPEARMINT LEAVES

⅛ PART LAVENDER FLOWERS

⅛ PART SLICED FRESH ORGANIC
ORANGES OR TANGERINES*

Make an infusion, following the directions on page 12.

To use: Enjoy 1–3 cups per day.

A pleasant and effective tea for headaches, muscle spasms, cramps, and other spazzy occasions. The hops is a bit bitter but is one of the important relaxing and antispasmodic herbs in this recipe, and it works well with the catnip and chamomile.

*Leave seeds and peel intact only if using organic fruit

Knockout-Drops Relaxing Tincture

1 PART FRESH VALERIAN ROOT

1 PART FRESH WILD LETTUCE

1 PART FRESH OR DRIED CHAMOMILE
FLOWERS

½ PART FRESH VALERIAN LEAVES
(OPTIONAL)

½ PART SLICED FRESH ORGANIC
ORANGES OR TANGERINES*

BRANDY

Make a tincture, following the directions on page 14.

To use: Take ½–1 teaspoon 1–3 times per day, as needed.

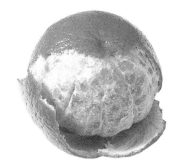

This is a potent tincture for relieving stress, insomnia, nervousness, anxiety, headaches, cramps, and muscle spasms. Fresh valerian is more effective than dried valerian root. You can also purchase ready-made valerian, wild lettuce, and chamomile tinctures and combine them in equal parts.

*Leave seeds and peel intact only if using organic fruit

Kava-Kava Dream Tea

I've been sharing this recipe with students and friends for years. A few of us discovered the relaxing and vivid dream-enhancing properties of kava-kava long before it became popular in the herb industry. Prepare the tea before bed, sip a nice hot cup, curl up with a good book, and see how long you can keep your eyes open!

2 PARTS KAVA-KAVA ROOT

1 PART CHAMOMILE FLOWERS

1 PART SKULLCAP LEAVES

1 PART PASSIONFLOWER LEAVES

1 PART WILD OATS

1 PART LEMON VERBENA LEAVES

1 PART ROSE HIPS

½ PART SPEARMINT LEAVES

Make an infusion, following the directions on page 12.

To use: Enjoy 1–3 cups per day. This tea is very nice with a touch of honey.

Easy-Does-It Relaxing Tea

This simple formula is wonderful before bed, and helps induce a peaceful and relaxed state. It can also be used throughout the day, to help you relax during stressful times. It's a gentle formula that tastes great hot or iced and can be drunk on a regular basis.

1 PART LEMON BALM (FRESH IF POSSIBLE)

1 PART LEMON VERBENA

1 PART LINDEN FLOWERS

1 PART WILD OATS

1 PART RED CLOVER BLOSSOMS

Make an infusion, following the directions on page 12.

To use: Take 1–4 cups per day, as needed.

Golden Slumber
Dreamtime Tea

2 PARTS ST.-JOHN'S-WORT

1 PART CHAMOMILE

1 PART WILD OATS

Make an infusion, following the directions on page 12.

To use: Take 1–2 cups before bedtime.

This tea is a pretty color, sort of a deep golden red-orange color. It helps you relax, and it induces vivid and colorful dreams. The quality of the St.-John's-wort is very important; if you are buying it dry, be sure it is bright green, not hay-like and pale, and also make sure there are plenty of bright yellow dried flowers mixed in with the leaves. This herb's active ingredients, hypericin and pseudohypericin, are in the flowers rather than the leaves.

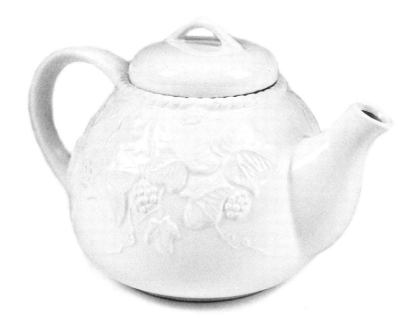

Kami McBride
VACCAVILLE, CALIFORNIA

Kami McBride's vision is to inspire a new culture that honors Earth and respects the female cycles of life. Her vision prompted the creation of the Living Awareness Institute, where she teaches an extensive herbal studies and women's health curriculum. Her most popular course, Cultivating the Herbal Medicine Woman Within, is an experiential study of the medicines of the earth and the healing wisdom of the female body.

An instructor of classes in herbal medicine and women's health since 1988, Kami teaches at many colleges and conferences in California, including the California Institute of Integral Studies Integral Health Department in San Francisco.

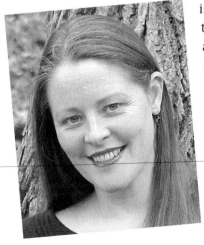

Kami is a sixth-generation resident of Vaccaville, California, and is blessed to have her home and consultation office located next to the creek where she grew up. Kami went on her first herb walk along that same creek when she was 8 years old. She remembers everything that was said about plant uses as she walked along the creek many years ago, and she feels that her deep connection with the land of her ancestors is at the heart of her herbal teachings. Kami's love for the earth was inspired by annual wilderness camping trips in the Sierras with her grandparents and seasonal family outings of foraging for wild food. She feels that working with plants helps establish a healing connection with Earth that is missing in so many people's lives. ✤

Kami's Avena Dreams Cordial

2 PARTS FRESH WILD OAT SPIKELETS
AND STRAW

BRANDY

1 PART PASSIONFLOWER LEAVES

1 PART FRESH ST.-JOHN'S-WORT
FLOWERING TOPS

HONEY

ROSE WATER

1. Harvest the top foot of green oatstraw while the pods are still milky (usually May–June). Mix in the passionflower leaves.

2. Cover with 2 times as much brandy. Let sit for 4–6 weeks.

3. Harvest fresh St.-John's-wort flowers. Cover with 2 times as much brandy, and let sit for 1 moon cycle (1 month) or 6 weeks.

4. Strain herbs from brandy. Add honey and rose water to taste, then combine tinctures.

To use: Take 1–2 droppersful 1–3 times per day, as needed.

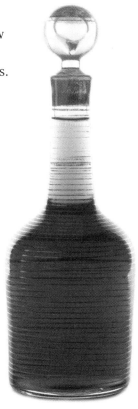

Kami recounts, "I have always lived in the golden rolling hills of California. Guess what is the golden part of those rolling hills? Oatstraw! Trampling through the oats since childhood, there is nothing more satisfying than using them as part of my favorite nerve tonic." Since St.-John's-wort flowers and oat seeds are usually harvested at different times (St.-John's-wort in June–July; oats in May–June), make each tincture separately, then add them together. This nourishing nervine tonic is great for soothing and tonifying a stressed-out nervous system.

Kami's Garden
Nerve Tonic Bath

Kami teaches a class called Healing through Beauty and Adornment, where herbal pampering is taken very seriously! Many herbal properties are absorbed through the skin, and herbal bathing therapies are powerful preventive medicine. For this reason, herbal bathing is one of Kami's favorite ways of toning and relaxing the nervous system, and she even includes an outdoor claw-foot bathtub situated on the edge of an oak forest as part of her classroom!

3 PARTS LAVENDER FLOWERS

2 PARTS LEMON BALM LEAVES

1 PART SKULLCAP LEAVES

1 PART BAY LEAVES

1 PART CALIFORNIA POPPY FLOWERS AND LEAVES (IF NOT AVAILABLE, SUBSTITUTE CHAMOMILE, CATNIP, OR HOPS)

1. Mix all ingredients. Put 2–3 cups of the mixture into a pot, and cover with 4 quarts boiling water.

2. Stir well, cover, and steep 15–20 minutes.

3. Strain out the herbs, and pour the tea into your bathtub. Immerse yourself, relax, and enjoy. Alternatively, you can prepare 2 quarts of this tea and use it to soak your hands or feet.

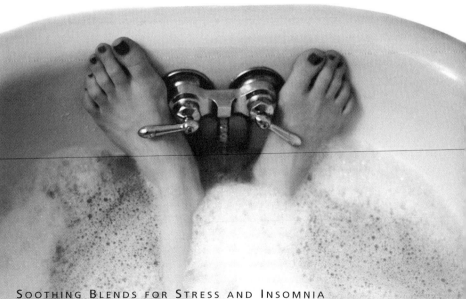

Athletic Endeavors: Performance Enhancers

Fresh-squeezed juices and nutrient-packed herbs and fruits are the key to the following recipes. How and what we consume before exercising significantly affects the way we feel during and after working out. The following recipes provide concentrated and balanced nutrients and antioxidants, both of which are important during aerobic exercise.

Herbal-a-Go-Go Morning Shake

Want to get up and go? Need something not too heavy but plenty energizing to enhance your workout routine? Tired of oatmeal and granola? Give this super shake a try. It has plenty of fresh nutrients and protein to give you a lasting boost.

YIELD: ABOUT 4 CUPS

2 CUPS FRESH ORANGE OR APPLE JUICE

1 CUP APRICOT OR STRAWBERRY YOGURT

1 CUP FROZEN MANGO OR BANANA CHUNKS

1 VIAL ROYAL JELLY

1 TABLESPOON BEE POLLEN

3 TABLESPOONS GROUND FRESH FLAXSEED (USE A COFFEE GRINDER TO GRIND THE FLAX)

¼ TEASPOON GROUND CARDAMOM POWDER

Place all ingredients in a blender. Blend well at high speed until smooth.

To use: Sip and enjoy half of the shake before your workout, and half after.

Strength and Stamina Ginseng Cordial

Ginseng has many well-proven benefits in boosting the body's ability to handle stress and exertion. It benefits the central nervous system and the muscles and stimulates the formation of healthy liver cells. This is a simple cordial to make and is very good to have on hand.

2 PARTS *PANAX* GINSENG ROOT

2 PARTS WHITE AMERICAN GINSENG ROOT

2 PARTS SIBERIAN GINSENG ROOT

2 PARTS HAWTHORN BERRIES

1 PART ROSE HIPS

1 PART LEMON VERBENA LEAVES

1 PART SARSAPARILLA ROOT

BRANDY

Make a cordial, following the directions on page 16.

To use: Enjoy ½–1 teaspoon 1 hour before workouts.

Flexibility Tea

3 PARTS NETTLE LEAVES

2 PARTS WILD OATS

2 PARTS HORSETAIL (STALKS)

1 PART ALFALFA LEAVES

1 PART BLUE ELDERBERRIES

1 PART HAWTHORN BERRIES

1 PART RED CLOVER BLOSSOMS

1 PART ROSE HIPS

¼ PART SLICED FRESH ORGANIC ORANGES OR TANGERINES*

This nutrient-rich blend nourishes and strengthens the ligaments, nerves, tendons, and bones. This mild-flavored tonic is appropriate to drink before or during a workout. This recipe can also be used to aid in sports injury recovery and in pre/post-surgery support.

*Leave seeds and peel intact only if using organic fruit

Make an infusion, following the directions on page 12.

To use: Enjoy 2–4 cups per day.

Blast-Off Herbal Smoothie

2 CUPS FRESH ORANGE, PINEAPPLE, OR APPLE JUICE

1 CUP STRAWBERRIES, FRESH OR FROZEN

1 CUP VANILLA FROZEN YOGURT OR VANILLA FROZEN RICE MILK (SUCH AS RICE DREAM)

¼ CUP CASHEW BUTTER OR ALMOND BUTTER

½ CUP CRUSHED ICE

2 TABLESPOONS VANILLA PROTEIN POWDER

1–2 TABLESPOONS SPIRULINA POWDER

This delicious smoothie has enough protein and nutrients to get you primed for a great workout. Spirulina works well in smoothies and is a definite nutrient boost. The smoothie will turn green from the spirulina; don't be alarmed!

YIELD: ABOUT 4 CUPS

Place all ingredients in a blender. Blend well at high speed until smooth.

To use: Sip and enjoy ½–1 hour before workouts. You can finish a leftover portion later in the day as well. Refrigerate any leftovers, and use within 2 days.

Revival Balls

These are definitely one of the most concentrated sources of herbal energy I know. They are rich in protein, calcium, magnesium, and iron and make a great treat for building up the blood and bones. I took these skiing the first time I made them, and I find they're incredible for an "instant revival" when you're cranking it out athletically. Try bringing some along on a backpacking or biking trip.

YIELD: ABOUT 60 BALLS

½ CUP RAW TAHINI

½ CUP ALMOND BUTTER OR CASHEW BUTTER

½ CUP HONEY OR BARLEY MALT SYRUP

½ CUP UNSWEETENED CAROB CHIPS

½ CUP CHOPPED, DRIED APRICOTS

3 TABLESPOONS BEE POLLEN

2 TABLESPOONS POWDERED DONG QUAI ROOT*

2 TABLESPOONS POWDERED *PANAX* GINSENG ROOT*

2 TABLESPOONS SPIRULINA POWDER

2 VIALS ROYAL JELLY

¼ CUP SESAME SEEDS OR SHREDDED COCONUT

1. In a bowl, stir together everything but the sesame seeds and coconut. Mix well.

2. Roll the mixture into little balls, about the size of small apricots.

3. Gently dry-roast ¼ cup sesame seeds or shredded coconut in a heavy-bottomed pan over low–medium heat, stirring constantly, until golden brown (about 1–2 minutes).

4. Roll the balls in the toasted coconut or sesame seeds. Store any leftovers in refrigerator; they will last for months.

To use: Enjoy just one or two as needed before, during, or after exercise. *Note:* Drink plenty of water with these; they are very concentrated.

*Purchase the dong quai and *Panax* ginseng in powdered form; they are very difficult to grind

The Happy Squeeze
Morning Smoothie

2 CUPS APPLE JUICE, FRESH-SQUEEZED
   OR FLASH-PASTEURIZED IF
   POSSIBLE

1 CUP VANILLA FROZEN YOGURT OR
   VANILLA FROZEN RICE DREAM

½ CUP FRESH OR FROZEN STRAW-
   BERRIES OR BANANAS

2–3 LARGE DATES, PITTED

2 TABLESPOONS VANILLA PROTEIN
   POWDER

2 TABLESPOONS ALMOND BUTTER
   OR PEANUT BUTTER

1 TABLESPOON BEE POLLEN

DASH CINNAMON

Place all ingredients in blender. Cover and
blend on high speed until smooth.
Refrigerate any leftovers;
they will last for 1–2
days.

To use:
Enjoy 8–16 ounces
1 hour before
working out. Drink
the rest later in the
day, or save for the
next day.

*You promised yourself
you'd get up and go to
the gym first thing in the
morning . . . but oh, your
warm bed feels so very
comfortable, and oh,
your mind is full of rea-
sons why it's not really so
important to get up after
all. Well, throw back
those covers, march into
your kitchen, and get
ready for the Happy
Squeeze — it's guaran-
teed to wake you up and
get you going!*

YIELD: ABOUT 4 CUPS

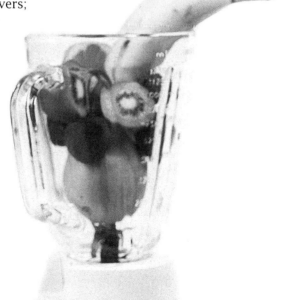

Susanne Paynovich
TIBURON, CALIFORNIA

Susanne Paynovich, B.A., is the owner of Waterborne Enterprises and creator of WaterGym, a deep-water aerobic workout. She is an aquatics-exercise specialist with 15 years' experience teaching, training instructors, and designing WaterGym workouts and equipment. She is ACE and AEA certified, is a yoga model, and has an extensive background in dance, sports, nutrition, and swimming.

For many years, Susanne (on the right in photo, with me) taught 20 or more WaterGym classes per week. The intense physical demand of teaching and running a rapidly growing business helped her define which foods supported her health and energy levels and which foods were detrimental. During this time she created some of her favorite recipes for sustaining optimal physical vitality.

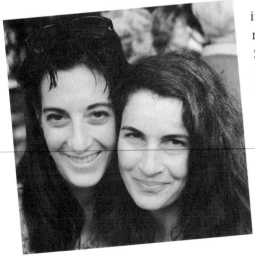

Susanne's earliest influences in the world of healthy cooking include Jack LaLane; Adele Davis; and Susanne's Italian mother, who could never feed her enough. In our early 20s, Susanne and I met in Santa Cruz, California. Together we worked in a gourmet natural foods restaurant, where we were often found tripping over the cooks in the kitchen, obsessed with creating exotic new recipes. To this day, Susanne still prefers four chocolate bars to fat-free yogurt, but luckily her talent as a healthy cook has kept her from succumbing to such desires.

To learn more about Susanne and her company, visit her Web site at www.watergym.com. ❦

Peachy Soy and Flax Shake

5 OUNCES TOFU

1 TABLESPOONS WHOLE FLAXSEEDS

¾ CUP COLD WATER

4 OUNCES FROZEN PEACHES (APPROXIMATELY 7 OR 8 PEACH SLICES)

2 TABLESPOONS FROZEN WHITE PEACH CONCENTRATE (WELCH'S IS GOOD)

Put all ingredients in a blender and blend until smooth. Refrigerate any leftovers; use within 2 days.

To use: Sip slowly over 1–3 hours while working around the house, or drink the entire amount 1 hour before a workout.

An energy-sustaining, blood sugar–stabilizing fruit shake, this unique drink is higher in protein, lower in carbohydrates, and not as sweet as commercial smoothies or shakes. Both the flax and the tofu give this shake a nutty taste and texture that will grow on you. Susanne says, "This is one of my favorite drinks to keep my mind sharp and my energy levels steady throughout the day."

YIELD: 1½ CUPS

Scrumptious Variations

When blended with water, tofu liquefies into a creamy, nutritious nondairy substitute for milk. Recent research has shown that isoflavones from soy help increase bone density and protect against certain cancers. The lignans and omega-3 oils from flax benefit the skin, reproductive organs, intestines, and heart.

If you loved flavored milk as a child, try a variation of the above recipe. Use frozen strawberries, mangos, blueberries, or bananas and less tofu so that the drink is thinner, like milk. Enjoy these fruity, nondairy milks as is, or pour them over cereal.

Susi's Sure-to-Cure-What-Ails-You Chicken Soup

According to Susanne, "This delicious, no-fuss soup has helped keep me healthy in the autumn–winter season. Whenever I'm coming down with a cold or flu, this nourishing soup has rapidly made me feel better." The formula will help induce a good sweat and chase away any "bugs."

YIELD: 4–5 SERVINGS

Making the Most of Your Soup

The medicinal properties of the garlic are crucial to the effectiveness of this soup. Raw garlic induces a sweat, which seems to burn the "evil" out of your cold. But beware, it will also scare away your friends! The Parmesan cheese makes the soup extra delicious, but leave it out if you have a cold or sore throat.

2 POUNDS ORGANIC CHICKEN

3 QUARTS WATER

3 STALKS OF CELERY, CHOPPED

2 MEDIUM CARROTS, CHOPPED

1 RED OR YELLOW ONION, SLICED

CHOPPED FRESH ZUCCHINI, YAMS, OR VEGETABLES OF CHOICE (OPTIONAL)

SALT OR TAMARI TO TASTE

1 BUNCH FRESH SPINACH, CHARD, KALE, BOK CHOY, OR COLLARD GREENS, WASHED AND CHOPPED

1½ TEASPOONS TAMARI

2 TABLESPOONS SWEET VERMOUTH (OR SHERRY OR MARSALA)

10 CLOVES FRESH GARLIC, CHOPPED

¼ CUP PARMESAN CHEESE

1. Wash chicken well. Remove skin and excess fat.

2. In a large soup pot, place the chicken in the water and bring to a boil. Boil rapidly for 3 minutes.

3. Reduce heat and simmer for 30 minutes, stirring occasionally.

4. Add the celery, carrots, onion, and other optional vegetables, and simmer another 15 minutes. Season lightly with salt or tamari.

5. About 5 minutes before the soup is done, wilt the fresh greens in a sauté pan with ¼ cup of the soup broth, stirring just until greens are lightly cooked, about 3–5 minutes.

6. Stir in 1½ teaspoons tamari and sweet vermouth.

7. Strain out the excess liquid from the greens, and pour it back into the soup.

8. Ladle soup into bowls. Top each bowl with a hearty serving of greens, a sprinkle of chopped fresh garlic, and Parmesan cheese.

Structural Healing: Recovery Tonics

If you have time to prepare for surgery, herbs and nutrients can be extremely helpful. Through their flavonoids, vitamins, and minerals, herbs help minimize trauma to the body and expedite healing of the injured area. In the case of unplanned surgery or a structural injury, herbs and good nutrition can still be used in the postoperative and recovery phases. I have personally seen great results with many people over the years, and I find that people respond well to the supportive nature of these recipes.

5 Favorite Flavonoids
Nourishing Tea

*Bioflavonoids and vita-
min C work hand in
hand to help strengthen
capillaries, cells, and tissues, and they are inti-
mately involved in
healing from injury.
Flavonoid-rich tonics are
helpful before and after
surgery or when some-
one is recovering from
injuries of any sort. This
tea is tasty and can be
drunk freely to assist
structural integrity and
healing.* Caution: *Ginkgo
acts as a blood thinner,
so leave it out of the
recipe for the 2 weeks
prior to surgery.*

1 PART CALENDULA BLOSSOMS

1 PART SLICED FRESH ORGANIC
    ORANGES OR TANGERINES*

1 PART GINKGO LEAVES

1 PART HAWTHORN BERRIES

1 PART ROSE HIPS

Make an infusion, following the directions on page 12.

To use: Enjoy 2–4 cups per day.

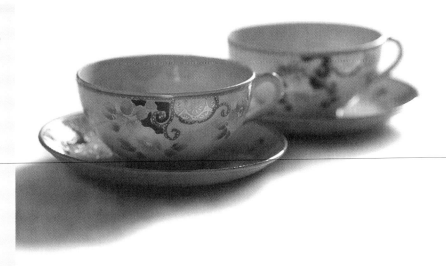

*Leave seeds and peel intact only
if using organic fruit

Simple Rose Hips Conserve

2 CUPS HOT WATER

1 CUP DRIED ROSE HIPS, CUT AND
   SIFTED (SEEDLESS)

½ CUP HONEY

2 TABLESPOONS FRESH LEMON JUICE

1 TABLESPOON VANILLA EXTRACT

1 TEASPOON POWDERED CINNAMON

This is absolutely delicious and can be made with dried rose hips. It's hard to keep enough of it around, so make plenty. It's always nice when a tonic that's so good for you tastes this good, too! This conserve is loaded with vitamin C and bioflavonoids, which aid in structural integrity and healing.

1. Pour the hot water over the rose hips in a bowl. Stir well, cover, and let sit for 1 hour.

2. Scoop the rose hips into a blender, using about half of the soaking water. Reserve the rest of the soaking water separately.

3. Add the rest of the ingredients into the blender. Blend well, until thick and puddinglike, adding more of the soaking water as needed.

4. Strain by stirring a little at a time through a large strainer. Scrape the conserve off the bottom outside surface of the strainer as needed. Straining the conserve will catch any stray seeds. (Cut and sifted rose hips, even though they say "seedless," always have a few seeds lurking in them. These seeds are very hard and can break a tooth, so be sure to strain your conserve!) Refrigerate conserve; it will last about 1 week.

To use: Spread on scones, muffins, pancakes, and waffles, or use as a topping for fruit salad or yogurt. Also great by the spoonful for colds, coughs, and sore throats. It's a great-tasting tonic for people of all ages.

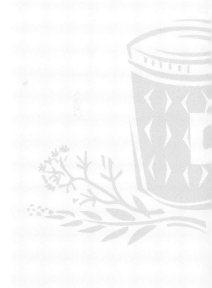

Calendula–St.-John's-Wort
Topical Healing Oil

This is a soothing, anti-inflammatory, external oil that is wonderful for helping heal burns, wounds, skin abrasions, and surgical incisions. It helps prevent scarring and really speeds up the healing process. It also works great on animals; I've used small amounts very successfully on kitty and doggy wounds. All of the ingredients are readily available at most natural foods stores or herb stores.

YIELD: 3 OUNCES

1 OUNCE FRESH CALENDULA FLOWER OIL

1 OUNCE FRESH ST.-JOHN'S-WORT OIL

1 OUNCE PURE VITAMIN E OIL (14,000 I.U.s)

1 TEASPOON PURE ESSENTIAL OIL OF LAVENDER (USE ½ TEASPOON IF THE FORMULA IS INTENDED FOR PETS OR PEOPLE WITH SENSITIVE SKIN)

1. In a clean paper cup or small plastic container, mix all ingredients together, stirring well. Pour the mixture into a clean 4-ounce glass bottle or plastic squeeze bottle. *Note:* Use a container that is just big enough to hold the oil; too much air in the container will cause the oil to degrade more quickly.

2. Store in a glass bottle in a cool dark place; it will last for a year or so.

To use: Apply sparingly several times per day to small areas such as cuts, scrapes, burns, bruises, or incisions. This formula also makes a fantastic facial oil for dry or sensitive skin; use just a few drops. Avoid getting the oil in the eyes, nose, or mouth.

A Versatile Remedy

The above oil is incredibly softening and nourishing for dry skin; it's superb as a facial oil or for under the eyes, on hands, on feet, on elbows, and more. It's a beautiful deep reddish orange color and smells wonderful, too!

Supple Sinews Turmeric–Ginger–Rose Hips Glycerite

1 PART GRATED FRESH GINGERROOT

1 PART ROSE HIPS

1 PART TURMERIC, FRESH OR DRIED

GLYCERIN

DISTILLED WATER

1. Place herbs in a widemouthed jar. If using fresh herbs, cover with 3 times as much glycerin. If using dry herbs, for every cup of base needed use ⅔ cup glycerin and ⅓ cup water. The total amount of base should be 3 times as much as the total amount of herb mixture.

2. Cover jar, and shake daily for 2 weeks.

3. Strain well. Compost herbs and rebottle the tincture.

To use: Take ½–1 teaspoon 2–3 times per day for acute injuries. As a tonic, take 1–2 teaspoons per day, several days per week.

This colorful nonalcoholic tincture draws upon the flavonoid-rich and anti-inflammatory properties of turmeric, ginger, and rose hips. Flavonoids assist in collagen formation, which is essential to healthy joint, nerve, and muscle tissue. It's a great formula for athletes, dancers, and anyone else who uses their sinews and muscles a lot. Glycerin is the perfect base for this tincture: It turns out sweet, spicy, and a gorgeous deep orange–red color.

Other Great Recipes

Many of the other recipes in this book are useful for structural healing. Try:

❋ Neen's Amazing Blood Building Soup (page 23) for an iron-rich, hearty, deeply nourishing, and immune-tonifying treatment

❋ Min-Elix Herbal Syrup (page 21) for a calcium-, magnesium-, and iron-rich, very deeply tonifying and blood-enriching recipe

❋ Hawthorn–Ginkgo Heart–Brain Tonic (page 54) for a flavonoid-rich, nourishing drink that will help heal injured tissues

❋ Flexibility Tea (page 103) for a mineral- and flavonoid-rich tonic that nourishes nerves, bones, ligaments, and more

Rasa Samanov and Michael Amster

IRVINE, CALIFORNIA

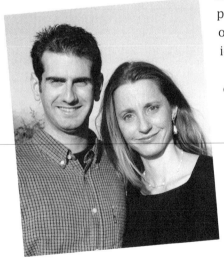

asa Samanov and Michael Amster are herbal soul mates who met at the American School of Herbalism in Santa Cruz, California. Their relationship is strengthened by a connection to plants and the study of the healing arts. Rasa and Michael are getting married in June 2000 and will be honeymoon-backpacking around the world, studying native healing traditions. Look for their integrative medical clinic in northern California following their return.

Rasa has been cultivating her love of plants since 1984. She spent over 7 years living intimately with the plants of the Big Sur wilderness. She completed a 5-year apprenticeship in traditional Chinese medicine with dear friend and teacher Lesley Tierra. Rasa is a nationally certified and California-state–licensed acupuncturist and currently practices in an integrative clinic with a medical doctor, naturopath, and midwife in Newport Beach. She teaches oriental medicine at University of California at Irvine's College of Medicine.

Michael became interested in herbalism as a premed student, while taking one of my introductory herbology classes. The course transformed Michael's understanding of healing and the holistic nature of health. While applying to medical school, Michael worked for 2 years as a researcher and assistant writer for Christopher Hobbs. Michael continues to integrate herbalism and alternative medicine as a 4th-year medical student at the University of California at Irvine and wishes to specialize in holistic family medicine. ⊕

Tonic Immune-Strengthening Congee

½ CUP BASMATI OR WHITE RICE (BROWN RICE OR OTHER GRAINS CAN ALSO BE USED)

3–4 CUPS FILTERED WATER, DEPENDING ON DESIRED THICKNESS

2 MEDIUM PIECES ASTRAGALUS ROOT (HUANG QI)

2 MEDIUM PIECES CODONOPSIS ROOT (DANG SHEN)

4 PIECES WILD YAM (SHAN YAO)

5 PIECES JUJUBE DATE (DA ZAO)

3 PIECES LICORICE ROOT (GAN CAO; OPTIONAL)

1–2 TABLESPOONS LYCII BERRIES (GOU QI ZI)

1. Rinse rice and combine with water in a rice cooker (with a porridge setting) or slow cooker. If cooking on the stove, combine the rice and water in a saucepan over low heat.

2. If using a rice cooker or slow cooker, add the herbs and allow to cook overnight. If cooking on the stove, add the herbs and stir occasionally over low heat until the grains are broken down (usually 4–6 hours).

3. When finished, remove the astragalus; it is too woody to eat. The softer herbs (lycii berries, jujube dates) can be left in the congee.

To use: Enjoy a morning bowl of congee 2–3 times per week in the autumn–winter season. If you're feeling weak or ill, eat daily as often as desired.

Congee is a dilute porridge usually made with rice (or other grains) and traditional Chinese tonic herbs. It is a slow-cooked, easily digested tonic and is the traditional food eaten in China for breakfast. Rasa recommends this valuable tonic to prevent disease and promote health. Congee is especially useful for people recovering from illness or surgery and is used in the treatment of poor digestion and low appetite, weakness, tiredness, depression, and lowered immunity.

YIELD: 2–3 CUPS

Bubbie's Miso–Chicken Soup

Michael's recipe for chicken soup combines the best wisdom of Jewish and Eastern traditions. For countless generations, Jewish grandmothers ("bubbies" in Yiddish) have cooked chicken soup for all types of ailments — most notably the common cold. Chicken soup is a vital part of Jewish culture, traditionally served every Friday night as "spiritual tonic" before the Sabbath meal and rituals. A traditional Jewish chicken soup with miso is an excellent meal to tonify the body and spirit.

YIELD: 2 QUARTS;
4–6 SERVINGS

1 MEDIUM-SIZED ONION

5 STALKS OF CELERY

4 CARROTS

2 TEASPOONS OLIVE OIL

2 TEASPOONS TAMARI

¼ CUP CHOPPED PARSLEY

1 TABLESPOON MIXTURE OF BASIL, ROSEMARY, THYME, AND OREGANO

1 BAY LEAF

3 QUARTS FILTERED WATER

1 POUND OF ORGANIC FREE-RANGE CHICKEN WITH THE BONES

5 CLOVES OF GARLIC, CHOPPED

2–3 TABLESPOONS LIGHT MISO MIXED WITH 1 CUP WARM WATER

TAMARI OR CELERY SALT TO TASTE

1. Slice onion, celery, and carrots. Heat oil and tamari in a large soup pot. Combine vegetables and herbs, and sauté in the oil for 5 minutes.

2. Add 3 quarts water, increasing heat to a boil.

3. Wash and skin chicken. Add to boiling water. Reduce heat and simmer for 2 hours.

4. Add chopped garlic and miso broth and remove from heat. Remove bay leaf. Add tamari or celery salt to taste. Refrigerate left-over soup; use within 4 days.

To use: Enjoy a steaming bowlful whenever you feel the need to nourish and fortify your body and soul.

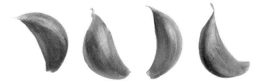

Mystic Herbals

Here we have it, the chapter you've been waiting for: love tonics, mystery potions, dream blends, sensory enhancers, nonalcoholic party drinks, and more. And each one is healthy, nourishing, flavorful, and so very fun to prepare and ingest. Over the years, I have seen numerous herbal students and friends get quite giddy over these recipes. They are scrumptious drinks to celebrate with, relax with, and get dreamy with. Many of these recipes are my absolute favorites of favorites: potions that have marvelous colors and flavors and just seem to hold a little magic in each bottle!

Love Potion #9 Herbal Cordial

This delicious cordial has had many incarnations over the years. I vary it each spring, and then enjoy it each summer, fall, and winter. It truly is a "mystic" that fulfills many roles: a delightful kissing potion, a heart/circulation tonic, and a vitamin C–rich winter tonic.

*Leave seeds and peel intact only if using organic fruit

3 PARTS ROSE HIPS

2 PARTS HAWTHORN BERRIES

2 PARTS HAWTHORN LEAVES AND FLOWERS

1 PART FRESH OR FROZEN STRAWBERRIES

1 PART FRESH OR FROZEN RASPBERRIES

1 PART SLICED FRESH ORGANIC ORANGES OR TANGERINES*

1 PART FRESH, RIPE, MASHED PERSIMMON OR MANGO

½ PART GRATED FRESH GINGERROOT

⅛ PART CINNAMON CHIPS

BRANDY

HONEY OR MAPLE SYRUP

Make a cordial, following the directions on page 16.

To use: Enjoy 1 teaspoon–1 tablespoon per day, several days a week, as a nourishing tonic for the heart and circulation. For special occasions, take up to 2 tablespoons as desired. For colds, coughs, and sore throat, take 1 teaspoon 3 times per day.

Moonlighting Tea

A colorful and flavorful blend for enhancing those cozy, romantic occasions, this tea is a nice, balanced blend of herbs to soothe, tone, and enhance your nerves and sensory system. It's wonderful hot or iced with a romantic picnic!

*Leave seeds and peel intact only if using organic fruit

2 PARTS DAMIANA LEAVES

1 PART CHAMOMILE FLOWERS

1 PART LEMONGRASS LEAVES

1 PART WILD OATS

1 PART PEPPERMINT LEAVES

1 PART ROSE HIPS

¼ PART JASMINE FLOWERS

¼ PART SLICED FRESH ORGANIC ORANGES OR TANGERINES*

⅛ PART LAVENDER FLOWERS

Make an infusion, following the directions on page 12.

To use: Enjoy 1–3 cups per day.

Fennel–Angelica
Fresh Summer Cordial

¼ CUP FRESH RIPE ANGELICA SEEDS*

2–3 CUPS CHOPPED FRESH FENNEL LEAVES, STALKS, AND FLOWERS

3–4 CUPS WATER

JUICE OF 3–4 FRESH LEMONS OR 5–6 LIMES

HONEY OR MAPLE SYRUP

FRESH EDIBLE FLOWERS OF CHOICE, SUCH AS JOHNNY-JUMP-UPS, PANSIES, BACHELOR'S BUTTONS, CALENDULA PETALS, ROSE PETALS, ROSE GERANIUM FLOWERS, OR BORAGE FLOWERS

1. Place the angelica seeds, fennel, and water in a blender. Cover, and blend well at high speed for 1 minute, until the herbs are liquefied and the cordial is bright green.

2. Strain out herbs through a fine strainer. Discard herbs, and reserve the bright green liquid.

3. Add the lemon or lime juice, and sweeten to taste. Serve in a pretty punch bowl, with plenty of ice cubes, and garnish with a few sprinkles of edible flowers.

To use: Enjoy a chilled wineglassful with a meal or by itself.

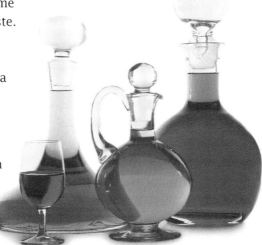

This exotic, nonalcoholic cordial is refreshing and digestive, and it captures the rapture of summer in a most unusual way. Angelica has much magic and folklore associated with it and seems to really make people giddy. It's especially enjoyable when sipped outdoors in a beautiful garden with good friends and good food. Note: *Angelica has a few deadly look-alikes; be sure you are using* Angelica archangelica. *Never ingest any herbs that you can't posiively identify.*

YIELD: 1½ QUARTS

*Do not use during pregnancy.

Tummy Love Wine

This was a spontaneous endeavor on a warm summer night in 1997; I was teaching a really fun 10-month herb course, and this was one of our herbal creations for a dinner party. We were divinely inspired to make an "old-fashioned" infused herbal digestive wine, and this was what we came up with. This is an especially nice recipe to make with fresh garden herbs and fresh summer fruits.

YIELD: 1 QUART

1 750-ML BOTTLE OF WHITE ZINFANDEL OR GEWURTZTRAMINER WHITE WINE

¼ CUP FRESH LEMON BALM LEAVES*

¼ CUP FRESH LEMON VERBENA LEAVES*

¼ CUP FRESH STRAWBERRIES

¼ CUP FRESH WATERMELON

¼ CUP ROSE HIPS, FRESH OR DRIED

2 TABLESPOONS FRESH FENNEL LEAVES

2 TABLESPOONS GRATED FRESH GINGERROOT

1 TABLESPOON FRESH ROSE GERANIUM BLOSSOMS*

A FEW SLICES FRESH ORGANIC ORANGE OR TANGERINE**

2 TEASPOONS CINNAMON CHIPS

1. Place all ingredients in a widemouthed glass jar. Cover and shake well.

2. Let sit overnight.

3. Refrigerate and continue to steep for 1 week–1 month.

4. Strain, rebottle wine, and keep in refrigerator. It will last for several months.

To use: Enjoy a chilled glassful with meals or with dessert.

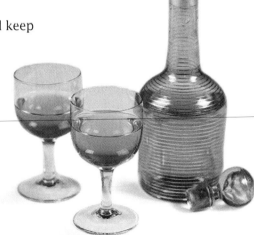

*Use dried if the fresh herbs are not available

**Leave seeds and peel intact only if using organic fruit

Instant Kiss Euphoria Honey

½ CUP HONEY

1 DROP PURE ESSENTIAL OIL OF ROSE GERANIUM*

1 DROP PURE ESSENTIAL OIL OF LEMON VERBENA*

1. Place the honey in a clean glass jar. Add the essential oils.

2. Stir well, then let the jar sit open for an hour or so, to let the flavors blend and mellow.

3. Store at room temperature in a covered jar; it will last indefinitely.

To use: Enjoy on warm, buttered sourdough bread or on scones, muffins, or toast. Also great in mint tea or chamomile tea, instead of plain honey.

This aromatic floral honey takes about an hour to make and can definitely bring on many compliments. It's been known to cause unexpected kissing, too; and as one of my students once said of this recipe, "It can make a man propose!"

YIELD: ½ CUP

*Available in natural foods or herb stores. *Caution:* Use *only* 1 drop of each essential oil, and be sure you are using pure, undiluted, food-grade essential oils

Rosie's Favorite Dream Tea

2 PARTS ST.-JOHN'S-WORT FLOWERS

½ PART NETTLE LEAVES

½ PART ROSE GERANIUM FLOWERS

½ PART SPEARMINT

Make an infusion, following the directions on page 12.

To use: Enjoy 1–2 cups before bedtime.

This recipe is simple but oh-so-effective for relaxing and soothing you into a deep and peaceful sleep and enhancing beautiful vivid dreams. My dear friend Rosie made this magical brew for me.

Stephanie Di Pietro
Scott's Valley, California

Stephanie Di Pietro, L.Ac., is the founder of Oriental Healing Arts, in Scott's Valley, California. She is an acupuncturist and herbologist with over 15 years of clinical practice. Stephanie specializes in functional medicine, applied nutrition, and orthopedics. She is a member of the American Association of Nutritional Consultants, the California Acupuncture Association, and the National Board of Acupuncture Orthopedics.

In her years of clinical experience, Stephanie has seen profound results from the proper use of acupuncture and herbal medicine. Her continued success in helping her patients to achieve their health goals is her greatest source of inspiration.

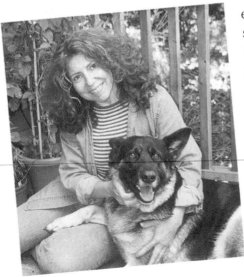

When asked to recall a significant personal herbal experience, Stephanie relates her story of being an acupuncture student under a great deal of stress, which caused her hair to turn rapidly and prematurely gray. Her teacher continually prescribed Chinese tonic herbs to nourish her chi and blood. It was quite impressive and dramatic when Stephanie's hair returned to its rich auburn color — in a mere three months!

Stephanie is conscientious and committed to helping others improve their health and well-being. Stephanie maintains a thriving practice in Santa Cruz County and the San Francisco Bay area. She is also one of the most creative and incredible gourmet cooks on the planet. Stephanie and I are close friends, and we delight in sharing outrageous multi-course meals together! ☙

Aphrodite's Oyster-Artichoke Soup

24 OUNCES FRESH, JARRED, OR CANNED
   OYSTERS, DRAINED (RESERVE LIQUID)

14 OUNCES ARTICHOKES, DRAINED

1 CUP WHITE WINE (OPTIONAL)

1–3 TABLESPOONS CHOPPED ITALIAN
   PARSLEY*

1 TEASPOON DRIED THYME*

2–6 STALKS OF CELERY

CAYENNE PEPPER TO TASTE

1 CUP CHOPPED VIDALIA ONIONS

1–2 CUPS 2-PERCENT LOW-FAT MILK

1–2 TEASPOONS GHEE OR OLIVE OIL

¼ CUP CHOPPED SCALLION GREENS

24 OUNCES CLAM JUICE

GROUND PEPPER TO TASTE

CHOPPED CHIVES, FOR GARNISH

1. Combine drained oysters and artichokes with white wine, and add the parsley and thyme.

2. Into a separate saucepan, pour all but ¼ of reserved oyster liquid. Add the chopped celery, cayenne pepper, and half of the onion. Simmer until vegetables are tender.

3. Let stock cool, then place in a blender or food processor and make a dense puree.

4. In the soup pot, melt the ghee. Add chopped green scallions and the other half of the onion; sauté 3 minutes or so.

5. Add the remaining oyster juice, clam juice, and spices; bring to a boil, then reduce heat and simmer, uncovered, for 10 minutes.

6. Add milk mixture to soup and stir continuously. Add the stock mixture, and add the oysters and artichokes. Cook until piping hot and until the oysters curl a little. Garnish soup with chopped chives.

To use: Serve with a nice salad and warm, crusty loaf of sourdough bread, by candlelight, to someone you adore.

Light the fire of your heart's desire with Stephanie's heart-healthy, mineral-rich, low-fat, creamy, and sumptuous soup; several of the ingredients have historically been considered aphrodisiacs. The soup can stand alone with a loaf of crusty bread and salad, or it can work well as a prelude to the delectables yet to come. Leftovers will keep well for 4–5 days if fresh ingredients are used and the soup is stored properly in the refrigerator.

YIELD: ABOUT 2 QUARTS

*For an exotic variation, use cilantro instead of parsley and thyme. Make a paste of smashed garlic clove, cilantro, jalapeño pepper, lemon juice, a small pinch salt, and a little curry; blend in blender until smooth

Shiitake–Tofu Paté

This is a delicious dip for marinated vegetables, or it can be diluted just a little and used as a rich sauce over brown rice and/or vegetables. Use high-quality organic tofu, and enjoy the benefits of soy protein, rich in isoflavones, which promote hormonal balance, strong bones, and a healthy heart. Shiitake is a delicious oriental mushroom that has immune-tonifying and cancer-preventing properties.

YIELD: 2 CUPS

1 SMALL ONION

3 OUNCES SHIITAKE MUSHROOMS

10 OUNCES FIRM, ORGANIC TOFU

2 TEASPOONS OLIVE OIL (OPTIONAL)

LIGHT, LOW-SALT TAMARI TO TASTE

SALT, PEPPER, OR CAYENNE TO TASTE

¼–½ CUP SALSA OF YOUR CHOICE
(PINEAPPLE SALSA IS A GOOD CHOICE)

½ TEASPOON FLAXSEEDS

1. Dice onion, mushrooms, and tofu.

2. Heat the oil in a sauté pan. Sauté the onion, shiitake mushrooms, and tofu, and add the tamari. Or in a nonstick pan, use the tamari for sautéeing, adding water if the pan gets dry. Sauté until the onions are translucent and the mushrooms are cooked.

3. Add a pinch of salt and pepper to taste (cayenne can be used if you like it spicy).

4. Put the sautéed ingredients in a blender along with the salsa, and puree to a smooth consistency. If it's too thick, add a little water or tamari, or even a little olive oil.

5. Put flaxseeds into a pepper grinder and, just before serving, grind them on top of the paté.

6. Mound the paté in the middle of a colorful assortment of fresh or marinated vegetables. Add some crackers to the outside of the plate. The paté can be served warm or chilled. It can be made a day ahead of time and will keep, refrigerated, for 3–4 days.

To use: Enjoy as a healthy, low-fat, immune-tonifying hors d'oeuvre.

Seasonal Tonics for Health and Good Cheer

And now, for the final festivities in the world of herbal tonics: holiday drinks and seasonal specials. What a fun note to end on! Whether it's hot or chilly outside, this chapter offers a beautiful array of recipes to brighten your day. Some of these recipes are easy to get "addicted" to, like a nice frosty glass of hibiscus cooler on a hot summer day. Or, on a cold winter night, how about steaming hot elder–lemon toddies? Never has it been so fun to help balance the weather patterns! Whatever the season, and whatever the weather, the following recipes are guaranteed to entice your taste buds and bring a smile to your face.

Hibiscus Cooler
Extraordinaire

This sun tea, which is made without boiling the water, is a gorgeous, deep magenta–purple, and the flavor is refreshing and tangy-sweet. The crimson hibiscus and rose hips are rich in natural vitamins A and C and electrolytes. Hibiscus Cooler is my drink of choice for long hikes, for backpacking trips, for picnics, and to take to the spa. It lasts well and can even be frozen and then defrosted slowly during long days in the sun.

3 PARTS HIBISCUS FLOWERS

2 PARTS ROSE HIPS

1 PART LEMONGRASS

1 PART CHOPPED FRESH RIPE PLUMS

1 PART SLICED FRESH ORGANIC ORANGES OR TANGERINES*

1/10 PART CINNAMON CHIPS

FRESH APPLE JUICE

PINEAPPLE JUICE

1. Place the fruit and herbs in a widemouthed glass jar. Cover with 4–5 times as much water, and stir well.

2. Place jar in sun for several hours, or place jar on counter and let sit overnight, until tea takes on a deep magenta color.

3. Strain and measure volume of tea. For every quart of hibiscus cooler, add 3 cups fresh apple juice and 1½ cups pineapple juice. (Color will change to a deep purple.) The tea will last for several days in the refrigerator, or freeze it and defrost it later.

To use: Enjoy by the glassful; or try freezing some in a bottle and then taking it with you on long bike rides, hikes, picnics, and other outings. Excellent during hot weather. This drink is also rich in electrolytes, making it a great choice for athletic endeavors.

*Leave seeds and peel intact only if using organic fruit

Ginger–Berry Cooler

⅓ CUP GRATED FRESH GINGERROOT

HONEY OR MAPLE SYRUP TO TASTE

1 QUART BLACKBERRY OR RASPBERRY JUICE

JUICE FROM 1–2 MEDIUM LEMONS (OPTIONAL)

1. In a large pot, boil 1 quart water. Add the ginger, reduce heat, and simmer, covered, for 10 minutes.

2. Turn off heat, and steep 10 minutes.

3. Strain, and sweeten lightly with honey or maple syrup to taste. Add the fruit juice, and lemon juice if desired, stir well, and freeze until slushy.

To use: Enjoy on hot days while the mixture is still slushy and semifrozen. Drink as much of this cold and spicy brew as you like.

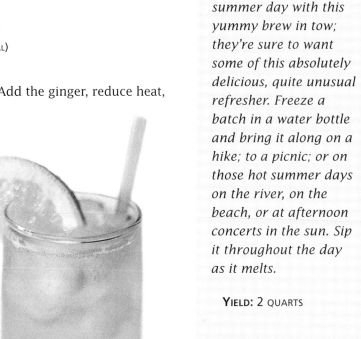

You can make many new friends on a hot summer day with this yummy brew in tow; they're sure to want some of this absolutely delicious, quite unusual refresher. Freeze a batch in a water bottle and bring it along on a hike; to a picnic; or on those hot summer days on the river, on the beach, or at afternoon concerts in the sun. Sip it throughout the day as it melts.

YIELD: 2 QUARTS

Caribbean Coolers

I invented this recipe on a warm summer night 20 years ago, at a tiny, tropical restaurant where I used to work. At that time chai was a little-known exotic tea that hardly anybody served. I decided to try making something a little different. Soon, people were coming in and ordering pitcherfuls.

YIELD: 3½ CUPS

2 CUPS COLD PREPARED CHAI, REGULAR OR DECAFFEINATED

1 CUP VANILLA DEAN ICE CREAM, VANILLA FROZEN YOGURT, OR FROZEN RICE MILK (SUCH AS RICE DREAM)

½ CUP CRUSHED ICE

A SPLASH COW'S, SOY, OR RICE MILK

1. Place all ingredients in a blender. Blend at high speed until thick and creamy, like a milkshake.

2. Serve in tall glasses, with colorful straws. Garnish glass with a slice of fresh orange.

To use: Enjoy a frosty glassful on a hot summer day or night. It's so delicious it will leave you wanting more!

Hot Brandied Elder–Lemon Toddies

These warming, relaxing, antiviral ingredients blend well into the old tradition of sipping hot toddies to dispel chills, coughs, and colds.

YIELD: ABOUT 12 OUNCES; 1 SERVING

*The red-berried variety is toxic; do not use

3 TABLESPOONS GRATED FRESH GINGERROOT

3 TABLESPOONS ELDER FLOWERS (FROM THE BLUE-BERRIED VARIETY)*

1 CUP BOILING WATER

⅛–¼ CUP BRANDY

JUICE OF 1 SMALL LEMON

2 TABLESPOONS HONEY

1. Prepare a tea of the elder flower and ginger by pouring boiling water over the herbs. Stir, cover, and allow to steep for 10 minutes.

2. Strain the tea, and pour into a large mug. Stir in the brandy, lemon, and honey.

To use: Sip slowly and enjoy.

Summer Blackberry–Nectarine Bliss

2 CUPS FRESH APPLE OR ORANGE JUICE

½ CUP FRESH OR FROZEN BLACKBERRIES

½ CUP FRESH OR FROZEN NECTARINE SLICES

½ CUP CRUSHED ICE

½ CUP FROZEN ORANGE SHERBET

1–2 DROPPERFULS FRESH ST.-JOHN'S-WORT TINCTURE OR GLYCERITE

1. Place all ingredients in a blender. Cover and blend well, until thick and smooth.

2. Refrigerate any leftovers; this will keep for 1–2 days.

To use: Sip a glassful slowly on a hot summer day, preferably while basking in the shade with a good novel or a close friend.

Caution on Drinking Toddies

Because of the relaxing effect of hot toddies, I usually recommend drinking them before bed, when you're at home and don't have to drive anywhere. If you leave the brandy out, you can drink these whenever.

This vitamin C–rich summer cooler is worth basking under a tree with; it's refreshing and nourishing and incredibly good on a hot summer day. If you have fresh blueberries or boysenberries, you can substitute them for the blackberries.

The St.-John's-wort adds a gentle nervine tonic quality to this formula, but remember that taking an herb occasionally is different from taking it every day in larger doses. St.-John's-wort was greatly publicized in 1998 for its anti-depressant effects, but it's also a gentle relaxant and nerve strengthener, and it blends well into this particular recipe.

YIELD: 4 CUPS

Holiday Crimson Cordial

This vitamin C–rich cordial is a delicious and useful holiday gift to help strengthen immunity and fight off winter ailments. It's nice to start a big batch in October or November and let it steep until just before Christmas.

*Leave seeds and peel intact only if using organic fruit

2 PARTS FRESH HAWTHORN BERRIES

2 PARTS FRESH ROSE HIPS

2 PARTS FRESH OR FROZEN RASPBER- RIES OR STRAWBERRIES

1 PART FRESH LEMON BALM

1 PART SIBERIAN GINSENG ROOT

1 PART GRATED FRESH GINGERROOT

1 PART SLICED FRESH ORGANIC ORANGES OR TANGERINES*

BRANDY

HONEY OR MAPLE SYRUP

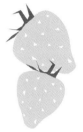

Make a cordial, following the directions on page 16.

To use: Take 1 teaspoon–1 tablespoon daily, a few days per week.

Peaches-and-Cream Summer Morning Smoothie

This is the taste of summer at its best. light, refreshing, and so very, very good. The delicate flavor of rose water adds just a touch of the exotic. You can also try orange blossom water for an equally delicious addition.

YIELD: 4 CUPS

2 CUPS FRESH ORANGE JUICE OR PINEAPPLE JUICE

1 CUP VANILLA OR PEACH FROZEN YOGURT

½ CUP FRESH OR FROZEN SLICED PEACHES

½ CUP CRUSHED ICE

½ TEASPOON PURE DISTILLED ROSE WATER

¼ TEASPOON PURE VANILLA EXTRACT

1. Place all ingredients in a blender. Cover and blend well.

2. Refrigerate any leftovers; this will last for 1–2 days.

To use: Enjoy a large glassful in the morning or afternoon as a refreshing, light meal.

Merry Magenta Herbal Punch

1 QUART WATER

½ CUP HIBISCUS FLOWERS

½ CUP ROSE HIPS

½ CUP SLICED FRESH ORGANIC ORANGES OR TANGERINES*

1 CINNAMON STICK, BROKEN INTO PIECES

½ TEASPOON WHOLE CLOVES

1 QUART CRANBERRY JUICE

2 CUPS PINEAPPLE JUICE

2 CUPS FRESH ORANGE JUICE

ICE CUBES

FRESH ROSE PETALS AND CALENDULA BLOSSOMS

This healthy version of fruit punch is a conversation starter at parties and other festive occasions. It's refreshing, full of vitamins A and C, and very fun to drink. This recipe also provides natural fruit acids and electrolytes and is especially good in very hot weather and before or after athletic endeavors.

YIELD: 3 QUARTS

1. Boil the water, and pour over the herbs, fruit, and spices. Stir well, cover, and steep for ½ hour.

2. Strain, and pour liquid into a glass bowl.

3. Add the cranberry, pineapple, and orange juices.

4. Add the ice cubes, and garnish with a sprinkle of fresh rose petals and calendula blossoms.

To use: Enjoy 1–2 cups as a refreshing party drink, during picnics, or before and after athletic activity.

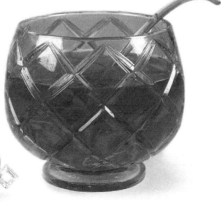

*Leave seeds and peel intact only if using organic fruit

Caitlin Adair
BRATTLEBORO, VERMONT

Caitlin Adair has been interested in herbs and wild plants of all kinds since childhood. She remembers enjoying the sweet nectar from clover blossoms on the lawn of her home in Illinois. In college, Caitlin bought her first pocket guide to wildflowers. She spent many delightful afternoons in nature, exploring the sweet wildness of Wisconsin. When she moved to Vermont in 1973, her interest in herbs for healing blossomed.

Caitlin's first herbal was Adele Dawson's *Health, Happiness and the Pursuit of Herbs.* Caitlin was inspired enough to seek out Adele, and they had a wonderful time visiting Adele's hillside garden and having tea together.

For years Caitlin has used herbs to treat family and friends. Mostly she just loves wild plants, enjoys knowing about them, and loves using them to help people. These days, Caitlin combines her passions into work with plants, houses, gardens, and people. She teaches a kind of natural T'ai Chi called the River. The River catches the energy of the place and the now-ness of the moment, promoting a deep and prayerful connection with the beauty of nature. It is like a beautiful slow-motion dance, a moving meditation that flows and changes like a river.

Among Caitlin's favorite herbs are damiana, a great tonic for the nervous system that is also said to be an aphrodisiac, and calendula. After seeing calendula growing wild on the island of Iona in Scotland, an ancient center of sacred learning for Druids as well as Christians, Caitlin developed a new appreciation for this common herb. ✤

Wise One's Tea

1 PART CHAMOMILE

1 PART DAMIANA

1 PART WILD OATS

1 PART ELDER FLOWERS (FROM THE BLUE-BERRIED VARIETY)

½ PART SAGE

Make an infusion, following the directions on page 12.

To use: Enjoy 2–4 cups per day.

Caitlin relates, "The herbs in this blend enhance our ability to access 'the wisdom archetype' within ourselves. This tea is a favorite in my kitchen."

Pagan Punch

1 PART CALENDULA FLOWERS

1 PART DAMIANA LEAVES

1 PART MEADOWSWEET (AERIAL PARTS)

1 PART RED CLOVER FLOWERS

1 PART SWEET WOODRUFF (AERIAL PARTS)

FRESH FRUIT JUICE

HONEY OR MAPLE SYRUP TO TASTE

FRESH CALENDULA FLOWER PETALS (OPTIONAL)

1. Make a strong infusion of herbs by following the directions on page 12, using 1–2 ounces of the mixture per quart of boiling water. (This can be done early in the day, or the day before you plan to serve it.)

2. Strain out the herbs. Add equal amount of fruit juice to the tea; cranberry and raspberry are good choices.

3. Sweeten lightly with honey or maple syrup to taste.

To use: Serve chilled, garnished with fresh edible flower petals of calendula if desired. Enjoy 1–2 cups per serving.

Says Caitlin, "I created Pagan Punch for Beltane, which is the celebration of Mayday, halfway between Spring Equinox and Summer Solstice. Beltane celebrates full flower and the dance of male and female. It is celebrated the world over with joy and merriment. Sweet woodruff, meadowsweet, and red clover all carry the energy of springtime and frolicking in flowery meadows."

YIELD: 2 QUARTS

Persian Rose Water Pudding

I love this mouth-watering dish. If you ever want to woo someone, this healthy, low-fat dessert qualifies as divinely inspiring in matters of love. It's quite exotic and a lovely treat for the body and soul. Rose water, cardamom, and vanilla are all traditionally associated with special occasions, feasting, and love.

YIELD: 4 CUPS

1 QUART LOW-FAT VANILLA YOGURT

2 TABLESPOONS HONEY

1 DROP PURE SWEET ORANGE ESSENTIAL OIL

1 TEASPOON PURE DISTILLED ROSE WATER**

¼ TEASPOON GROUND CARDAMOM

1 TABLESPOON FRESH ROSE PETALS

¼ CUP SLICED FRESH STRAWBERRIES OR WHOLE RASPBERRIES

1. Place a colander or strainer into a bowl. Line the colander or strainer with a couple of layers of cheesecloth. Gently scoop the yogurt into the colander.

2. Cover top of colander with a plate, and let sit in refrigerator overnight. This will thicken the yogurt by allowing the whey to drain out.*

3. The next day, gently scoop the yogurt into a pretty bowl, or onto a nice serving plate.

4. Mix the honey with the orange essential oil. Drizzle the honey, rose water, and cardamom over the yogurt.

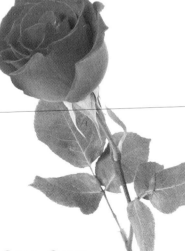

5. Garnish with fresh rose petals and fresh berries.

To use: Feed this by candlelight to someone you love!

*Save the whey: It's full of good nutrients and healthy acidophilus. Whey can be mixed into drinks and juice or drunk straight. It tastes good!

**Available in herb or natural food stores, as well as Greek or Mediterranean delis

A Materia Medica of Tonic Herbs

This chart gives a concise overview of most of the herbs used in the healing tonic recipes. For each herb, I've listed the common and botanical Latin names, the parts used, the general taste characteristics, the herb's properties and uses, and the herb's affinity for particular body systems. While by no means exhaustive, this list provides general knowledge about each herb so that you can familiarize yourself with the herbs and make informed decisions before using them in formulas. For further information, consult some good herb books, such as *The Illustrated Herb Encyclopedia* by Kathi Keville, *The Complete Book of Herbs* by Lesley Bremness, and *The Holistic Herbal* by David Hoffmann.

HERB	PART USED	TASTE	AFFINITY FOR	PROPERTIES	USE IN FORMULAS FOR
Alfalfa (*Medicago sativa*)	Leaves	Bland, pleasant, grassy	Entire system	Alterative; nutritive, rich in vitamins, protein, and minerals; antiarthritic	Increasing overall nutrition and vitality; alkalinizing the blood and cleansing excess uric acid from system; pre- and postnatal tonics
Angelica* (*Angelica archangelica*)	Root, stem, leaves	Spicy, aromatic, maplelike, bitter	Throat, lungs, stomach, uterus	Antiviral, warming, antispasmodic, digestive, emmenagogue	Colds, flu, coughs; digestion; menstrual cramps
Aralia (California spikenard, California ginseng) (*Aralia californica*)	Root	Spicy, carrotlike, maplelike, slightly bitter	Lungs, immune system	Warming, antiviral, adaptogenic, expectorant, demulcent, tonic	Strengthening lungs; fighting off colds, coughs; strengthening overall stamina and resistance
Astragalus (*Astragalus membranaceus*)	Root	Bland, sweet, woody	Immune system, lungs, spleen	Immune tonic; strengthens lungs and spleen; increases natural killer cells, T-helper cells, and interferon production	Enhancing immune system; pre- and postsurgical care; before, during, and after chemotherapy or radiation
Burdock (*Arctium lappa*)	Root	Earthy, nutritive, slightly bitter	Liver, kidneys, lymph, blood	Alterative, nutritive, antiarthritic, cleanses blood and lymph, tones liver	Sluggish digestion, elimination; skin problems; general cleansing and detox
Calendula (*Calendula officinalis*)	Flowers	Aromatic, slightly resinous, pleasantly medicinal	Skin, lymph, mucous membranes, spleen	Alterative, antiviral, bacterial, antifungal, demulcent, vulnerary, anti-inflammatory	Sore throat and swollen glands; internal or external irritations; wound healing, postsurgical scars

***Caution:** Do not use during pregnancy. In addition, if you're harvesting your own fresh angelica be absolutely positive in your identifications; this herb has many deadly look-alikes.

HERB	PART USED	TASTE	AFFINITY FOR	PROPERTIES	USE IN FORMULAS FOR
Chamomile (German, *Matricaria recutita*; Roman, *Anthemis noblis*)	Flowers	Slightly bitter, aromatic, astringent, applelike	Stomach and nerves	Antispasmodic, digestive, nervine, anti-inflammatory, mildly sedative	Indigestion; cramps and bloating; stress, nervousness, insomnia
Chickweed (*Stellaria media*)	Whole plant, preferably fresh or freshly dried	Mild, fresh, delicately green	Mucous membranes, blood, kidneys	Cooling, demulcent, vulnerary, anti-inflammatory, diuretic, nutritive; high in vitamins A and C, calcium, and iron	Healing internal or external irritations (including those of the kidney and bladder); building blood; PMS or menopause
Codonopsis (dang shen) (*Codonopsis pilosula*)	Root	Sweet, bland, pleasant	Lungs, spleen, immune system	Adaptogenic, demulcent, immune tonic	Increasing resistance and vitality; strengthening lungs and spleen; structural healing; pre- and postsurgical recovery, increasing strength and stamina; preventing jet lag
Dandelion (*Taraxacum officinale*)	Leaf and root	Bitter, earthy, nutritive	Liver, kidneys, blood	Alterative, diuretic, blood purifying, nutritive, tones liver and digestion	Congested or stagnant liver, digestion; skin problems; PMS and menopause
Dong Quai* (*Angelica sinensis*)	Root	Smoky, aromatic, maple-like, bitter	Blood and uterus	Builds blood and chi (life force), nutritive, regulates and balances female hormones, emmenagogue	Irregular menses; PMS and menopause; infertility or weak reproductive organs; anemia; low vitality

*Caution: Do not use during pregnancy.

HERB	PART USED	TASTE	AFFINITY FOR	PROPERTIES	USE IN FORMULAS FOR
Echinacea (*Echinacea purpurea, E. angustifolia*)	Root (leaves, flowers, and seeds also useful, although the root is thought to be the strongest)	Aromatic, produces a tingly sensation on the tongue	Throat, lymph and immune systems	Lymphatic, antiviral, antibacterial, alterative, enhances immunity	Acute or chronic infections; sore throat; building immune system; increasing resistance to upper respiratory infections
Elder (*Sambucus nigra, S. mexicana*)	Flowers, berries (from blue-berried variety only)	Berries: tart and fruity; flowers: delicate, floral, astringent	Lungs and upper respiratory system, especially sinuses and throat	Flowers are antiviral, diaphoretic, astringent; berries are rich in vitamins A and C and flavonoids, and they strengthen eyes, vascular system, and connective tissue	Colds, flu, coughs; cleansing and detox; skin problems
Fennel* (*Foeniculum vulgare*)	Fresh leaves and stalks; fresh or dried seeds or flowers	Sweet and aromatic, reminiscent of anise or licorice	Throat, lungs, and stomach	Antispasmodic, galactogogue (promotes the flow of milk in nursing mothers), carminative, soothing, demulcent, slightly estrogenic; good for lungs, throat, stomach	Coughs, colds, and sore throat; indigestion, gas and bloating; increasing milk flow in nursing mothers
Fenugreek** (*Trigonella foenum-graecum*)	Seeds	Aromatic and maplelike	Throat, lungs, stomach, and hormonal system	Mucilaginous, expectorant, galactogogue, anti-inflammatory, contains phyto-steroids	Sore throat and coughs; female tonics; cleansing digestive tract

*Caution: Do not use in large quantities if you have estrogen-dependent breast cancer. Do not use fresh seeds during pregnancy.
**Caution: Do not use in large quantities if you have estrogen-dependent breast cancer.

HERB	PART USED	TASTE	AFFINITY FOR	PROPERTIES	USE IN FORMULAS FOR
Flax (*Linum usitatissimum*)	Seeds	Bland and nutty	Mucous membranes, especially in the lungs, throat, intestines, and bladder	Mucilaginous, anti-inflammatory, nutritive (rich in omega-3 essential fatty acids)	Sore throat, irritated intestinal tract (as a tea); food supplement for essential fatty acids (as freshly ground seeds); supplement to support health of heart, hormonal system, and skin (as an oil or freshly ground seeds)
Garlic (*Allium sativum*)	Cloves	Warm and pungent, onionlike	Entire system, but especially the lungs and blood	Antiviral, antibacterial, antifungal, warming, expectorant, antihypertensive	Fighting off colds, flu, and systemic infections; helping lower cholesterol; warming and stimulating the digestive tract, lungs, and circulatory system
Ginger (*Zingiber officinale*)	Root	Aromatic, spicy, hot	Throat, lungs, stomach, circulatory system	Carminative, anti-inflammatory, circulatory stimulant, diaphoretic, antispasmodic	Colds, flu, coughs; sluggish digestion; poor circulation
Ginseng, Asian* (*Panax ginseng*)	Root	Aromatic, woody, earthy, maplelike, slightly sweet, bitter	Blood, circulatory system, immune system, endocrine system	Adaptogen, builds blood and chi, improves physical and mental performance; one of the best overall energy and endurance tonics	Increasing energy, mental clarity, and vitality; strengthening immunity; hormonal balancing; athletic endeavors; physical stress
Gotu Kola (*Centella asiatica*)	Whole plant	Bittersweet, acrid	Brain, nervous system, blood, reproductive organs	Tonic, blood purifying, anti-inflammatory, vulnerary, nervine	Brain tonics; nervous exhaustion; postoperative healing

***Caution:** Do not use if you are pregnant or nursing or have high blood pressure.

HERB	PART USED	TASTE	AFFINITY FOR	PROPERTIES	USE IN FORMULAS FOR
Hawthorn (*Crataegus oxyacantha, C. monogyna, C. laevigata*)	Leaves, flowers, berries	Leaves and flowers are pleasantly astringent, a little like green tea; berries are fruity, bland, soothing	Heart, circulatory system, connective tissue	Cardiotonic, strengthens entire cardiovascular system; flavonoid-rich; assists body in structural repair from injury and surgery; demulcent	Cardiovascular system; pre- and postsurgery; recovery from injury; restlessness and insomnia
Jujube Dates (*Ziziyphus jujuba*)	Fruit	Sweet and slightly smoky	Digestive tract, nerves, emotions	Mildly tonic for digestion and energy, mildly sedative	Building energy and vitality; poor appetite; nervous exhaustion; emotional stress
Kava-Kava* (*Piper methystichum*)	Root	Resinous, woody, bitter	Nervous system	Relaxing nervine, dream enhancing, slightly euphoric, antispasmodic	Insomnia, nervousness, stress; pain; menstrual cramps
Lavender (*Lavandula* spp.)	Flowers and leaves	Aromatic, floral, astringent	Nerves, muscles, skin	Antispasmodic, antiseptic, relaxing and uplifting nervine, cytophylactic (promotes formation of healthy skin cells), vulnerary, carminative	Nervous tension, tight muscles, insomnia, anxiety; skin, muscle, and nerve injuries (can be used topically and internally)
Lemon Balm (*Melissa officinalis*)	Leaves, preferably fresh or freshly dried	Aromatic, lemony, pleasant, refreshing	Stomach, immune system, nerves	Antiviral, carminative, uplifting and soothing nervine	Colds, flu, herpes, chicken pox; digestion; stress, insomnia, anxiety

*Caution: Do not use during pregnancy. Also, do not use on a daily basis; kava-kava is full of resinous lactones, which can be taxing on the liver and kidneys if overused.

HERB	PART USED	TASTE	AFFINITY FOR	PROPERTIES	USE IN FORMULAS FOR
Lemongrass (*Cymbopogon citratus*)	Leaves	Mildly lemony, very pleasant; good as a flavoring	Throat, stomach, nerves	Cooling, thirst-quenching, mildly carminative, relaxant	Cooling the body; digestive blends; relaxing blends; flavoring for bitter or less-tasty herbs
Lemon Verbena (*Aloysia triphylla*)	Leaves	Aromatic, exotic, lemony with a bit of vanilla, refreshing	Nerves, stomach	Uplifting nervine, carminative, cooling	Stress and anxiety; digestion; cooling the body; flavoring for bitter or less-tasty herbs
Licorice* (*Glycyrrhiza glabra*)	Root	Sweet, woody, aniselike	Lungs, throat, stomach	Demulcent, anti-inflammatory, rich in phytosteroids, mildly estrogenic	Irritation of throat and lungs; ulcers; female tonics; adrenal tonics; flavoring for bitter or less-tasty herbs
Lycii (*Lycium chinense*)	Berries; only the dried form is available commercially	Sweet, slightly smoky, raisinlike	Liver, blood, eyes, kidney	Nutritive tonic for blood, liver, and kidneys; rich in beta-carotene	Anemia; poor eyesight, blurred vision; sexual impotence; low energy or vitality
Meadowsweet (*Filipendula ulmaria*)	Aerial parts	Astringent	Gastric mucosa, rheumatic joints, lower bowel	Anti-inflammatory, anodyne, antipyretic, antacid, antiseptic-diuretic	Fever; pain; gastric ulcers; urinary tract infections; rheumatism
Mint (Peppermint, *Mentha* x *piperita*; spearmint, *M. spicata*)	Leaves	Refreshing, slightly menthol-like, astringent	Digestive tract	Carminative, astringent, diaphoretic	Indigestion, gas, bloating, stomach flu; flavoring for less-tasty herbs

*Caution: Do not use if you have high blood pressure or estrogen-dependent breast cancer.

Tonic Herbs and Their Uses

HERB	PART USED	TASTE	AFFINITY FOR	PROPERTIES	USE IN FORMULAS FOR
Motherwort* (*Leonurus cardiaca*)	Aerial parts	Bitter, astringent	Heart, uterus, nerves	Cardiac tonic, emmenagogue, antispasmodic, nervine	Heart tonics; delayed menstruation; nervous tension and anxiety; menopause
Mugwort* (*Artemisia vulgaris, A. douglasiana*)	Leaves, preferably fresh or freshly dried	Aromatic, sage-like, bitter	Liver, stomach, nerves, uterus	Digestive, carminative, nervine, emmenagogue, antispasmodic	Sluggish liver and digestion; reducing sweet cravings; reducing irritability associated with PMS; inducing menstruation in non-pregnant women.
Mullein (*Verbascum thapsus*)	Leaves	Mild and pleasant	Lungs	Demulcent, expectorant, tonic for lungs	Coughs; lung infections; strengthening upper respiratory tract
Nettle (*Urtica dioica*)	Leaves (preferably young and tender), stems	Pleasant, full-bodied, earthy	Blood, kidney, adrenals, reproductive system	Alterative, nutritive, blood building tonic for whole body	Anemia, blood building; low vitality; building strength and stamina; prenatal, postpartum, PMS, menopause; musculoskeletal healing, pre- and postsurgery
Orange** (*Citrus sinensis*)	Fruit, inner peel, outer peel	Fruit is sweet, juicy, citrusy; inner peel is bland; outer peel is aromatic, slightly bitter, citrusy	Lungs, throat (fruit and peel); vascular system (inner peel); stomach (outer peel)	Fruit is nutritive, cooling, refreshing, rich in vitamin C; outer peel is antiseptic, carminative, stimulates digestion; inner peel is rich in bioflavonoids, supports vascular system	Colds, flu, coughs (fruit and peel); sluggish digestion (fruit and peel); structural healing, pre- and postsurgery (fruit and inner peel)

* **Caution:** Do not use during pregnancy.

** **Caution:** Always use organic oranges (and other citrus fruits); commercial citrus fruits are heavily sprayed with pesticides.

HERB	PART USED	TASTE	AFFINITY FOR	PROPERTIES	USE IN FORMULAS FOR
Oregon Grape* (*Mahonia aquifolium* syn. *Berberis aquifolium*)	Root	Astringent, bitter,	Liver, blood	Hepatic, alterative, antiseptic, antibacterial	Liver and stomach; sluggish digestion; poor elimination; bacterial infections, especially of the stomach; skin problems such as acne, psoriasis, and eczema
Osha* (*Ligusticum porterii*)	Root	Aromatic, bitter, maplelike	Throat, lungs, uterus	Antiviral, antibacterial, warming, expectorant, emmenagogue	Chest colds and coughs; bronchial infections and pneumonia; delayed menses
Partridgeberry (*Mitchella repens*)	Aerial parts and berries	Slightly bitter	Uterus, ovaries	Uterine tonic, galactogogue, diuretic	Strengthening uterus, normalizing hormones; easing labor and delivery; increasing flow of breast milk in nursing mothers; easing heavy, painful menses
Passionflower (*Passiflora incarnata*)	Leaves	Slightly bitter, cooling	Nerves	Relaxing nervine, antispasmodic, mildly sedative	Nervous tension, anxiety, and insomnia; physical tension and pain
Red Clover** (*Trifolium pratense*)	Flowers	Sweet, pleasant, honeylike	Blood, lungs, skin, nerves	Alterative, blood purifying, nutritive, mildly antispasmodic, rich in phytoestrogens (may protect against certain cancers)	Nourishing and cleansing the blood; soothing coughs and colds; relaxing nerves; PMS and menopause; promoting health of reproductive organs

*Caution: Do not use during pregnancy.

**Caution: Do not use in large quantities if you have estrogen-dependent breast cancer.
Do not use 2 weeks prior to surgery.

HERB	PART USED	TASTE	AFFINITY FOR	PROPERTIES	USE IN FORMULAS FOR
Red Raspberry (*Rubus strigosus, R. idaeus*)	Leaves and fruit	Leaves are robust, astringent, a little like green tea; fruit is tart, juicy, berrylike	Uterus, mucous membranes	Tonic for uterus, astringent (leaves); rich in vitamin A and C, cooling, and thirst-quenching (berries)	Prenatal and postnatal tonics, PMS, menopause, astringent for the lower bowel (leaves); nutritious and flavorful addition to cordials, tinctures, and drinks (berries)
Rehmannia (shu di huang) (*Rehmannia glutinosa*)	Cooked root	Smoky, sweet like maple syrup or dried apricots, pleasant	Blood, kidney, adrenals, uterus	Blood building, tonic for kidneys, adrenals, uterus; hormonal balancing	Anemia and low vitality; PMS, menopause, irregular menses, infertility
Reishi Mushroom (*Ganoderma lucidum*)	Fresh or dried mushroom	Bland, pleasant, woody	Immune system, nerves, heart, adrenals	Tonifies immune system, calms nerves, nourishes heart	Boosting immunity; nervousness and anxiety; general weakness and fatigue; systemic support during chemotherapy and radiation treatment
Rose (*Rosa* spp.)	Petals and rose hips	Petals are floral, delicate, astringent; rose hips are tart and fruity	Skin (petals); throat, lungs, cardiovascular system (rose hips)	Rose petals, while not medicinal, are edible and tasty in delicate sauces, desserts, cordials, and drinks; rose hips are rich in bioflavonoids and vitamins A and C and are soothing and nutritive for the entire system	Cooling and nutritious summer drinks, colds, flu, coughs; structural healing: pre- and postsurgery; children's coughs and colds; great source of vitamin C
Rose Geranium (*Pelargonium graveolens*)	Leaves and flowers	Rosy and citrusy, astringent	Nervous system, skin	Uplifting, calming, refreshing, astringent	Summer coolers and lemonades; externally in skin and facial products; relaxing

HERB	PART USED	TASTE	AFFINITY FOR	PROPERTIES	USE IN FORMULAS FOR
Rosemary (*Rosmarinus officinalis*)	Leaves, flowers	Slightly piney and aromatic, resinous, pungent	Nerves, brain, skin, muscles	Tonic-nervine, antispasmodic, anodyne, antioxidant; contains salicin, a natural glycoside from which aspirin is made	Tired nerves, impaired nerve function; nerve or muscle tension and pain; headaches; fevers; flus; brain and memory tonics
Sage (Garden sage, *Salvia officinalis; S. tricolor;* California black sage, *S. mellifera*)	Leaves, flowers	Aromatic, slightly camphorlike, astringent	Lungs, liver, brain, nerves	Antibacterial, antiviral, astringent, diaphoretic, tonic-nervine	Colds, flu, coughs; fever, achy muscles; brain and memory tonics
Sarsaparilla (*Smilax* spp.)	Root	Sweet, woody, slightly vanilla-like	Liver, blood, glandular system	Alterative, blood purifying tonic for liver	Skin problems such as acne and eczema; sluggish digestion and elimination; male and female hormonal tonics
Saw Palmetto (*Serenoa repens*)	Berries	Pungent	Prostate, bladder, reproductive organs	Anti-inflammatory, diuretic, nutritive	Benign prostatic hypertrophy (BPH); chronic susceptibility to bladder infections in men or women; improving tone and health of bladder, prostate, and reproductive organs
Schisandra (*Schisandra chinensis*)	Berries	Sour, pungent	Liver, lungs, immune system	Adaptogenic, immune-tonic	Boosting immunity; adapting to stress; protecting liver; strengthening lungs
Shiitake Mushroom (*Lentinus edodes*)	Fresh or dried mushroom	Bland, pleasant, earthy	Immune system, liver	Immune-tonic, antineoplastic (cancer fighter), antiviral	Immune system; systemic support during chemotherapy and radiation treatment; environmental allergies; hepatitis, AIDS, *Candida* infections

HERB	PART USED	TASTE	AFFINITY FOR	PROPERTIES	USE IN FORMULAS FOR
Siberian Ginseng (*Eleutherococcus senticosus*)	Root	Bland, woody, pleasant	Adrenal glands, immune system, entire body	Adaptogenic; tonic for adrenals, memory, immune system	Mental clarity, memory enhancement; increasing energy and vitality; reducing jet lag, athletic activity and physical exertion
Skullcap (*Scutellaria lateriflora*)	Leaves	Slightly bitter, astringent	Nerves	Nervine, antispasmodic	Anxiety, stress, and insomnia; PMS and menopause; physical tension and pain; pain associated with herpes, shingles, and sciatica
St.-John's-Wort (*Hypericum perforatum*)	Flowering tops	Slightly sweet, astringent	Nervous system, connective tissue, skin	*Internally:* nervine, antidepressant, relaxant, antiviral; *externally:* anodyne, anti-inflammatory, vulnerary	Internally for anxiety, stress, insomnia, mild-to-moderate depression, nerve damage or weakness, herpes, shingles, and other Epstein-Barr–type viral infection; externally as an oil for burns and scrapes, nerve damage, pain, sciatica, dry or irritated skin
Thyme (*Thymus* spp.)	Leaves	Pungent, aromatic, spicy	Sinuses, throat, lungs, immune system	Antiviral, antibacterial, antifungal (great germicide)	Sinus, throat, and lung infections; systemic infections such as *Streptococcus* and *Staphylococcus*; gargle for sore throat
Usnea (*Usnea* spp.)	Whole lichen	Mossy, earthy, slightly astringent	Sinuses, throat, lungs, immune system, urinary tract	Antibiotic, antifungal, antiviral	Sinus, throat, and lung infections; bladder infections; *Candida* infections
Valerian (*Valeriana officinalis*)	Root	Aromatic, earthy, distinctive	Nervous system, uterus, musculoskeletal system	Nervine, sedative, antispasmodic	Anxiety, stress, insomnia; muscle tension and pain; menstrual cramps

HERB	PART USED	TASTE	AFFINITY FOR	PROPERTIES	USE IN FORMULAS FOR
Violet (Viola odorata)	Leaves, flowers	Bland, slightly like wintergreen	Blood, lymph, throat	Demulcent, expectorant, nutritive, alterative, cleansing, rich in vitamins A and C	Sore throat, cough, lung irritation; blood or lymphatic cleansing; nutritive whole-body tonic
Vitex (chaste berry) (Vitex agnus-castus)	Berries	Spicy, similar to black pepper	Endocrine system	Hormonal balancing, galactogogue	Balancing progesterone levels; PMS, menopause; certain types of uterine tumors and cysts; irregular menstrual cycles
Wild Oat (Avena sativa)	Straw (fresh or dried stem) and spikelets	Delicate, pleasant, slightly sweet, mild	Nerves, joints, tendons, bones	Nutritive (especially rich in calcium), nervine, antiaddictive	Nervous exhaustion, anxiety, insomnia; structural healing, pre- and postsurgical care; prenatal, postpartum, PMS, menopause
Yarrow (Achillea millefolium)	Flowers	Astringent, bitter	Sinuses, throat, lungs, skin, mucous membranes	Antiviral, antibacterial, diaphoretic, anti-inflammatory, astringent	Colds and flu; systemic infections; heavy, crampy menstruation; sore throat; tonsillitis
Yellow Dock (curly dock) (Rumex crispus)	Root	Pleasant, astringent, earthy, bitter	Liver, gallbladder, digestive tract, blood, skin	Blood purifying, alterative, digestive, nutritive (iron-rich)	Sluggish digestion and elimination; skin problems such as acne, eczema, psoriasis; anemia; tonics (high in iron, and also helps body absorb iron from other foods and herbs)
Yerba Santa (Eriodictyon californicum)	Leaves	Pleasant, resinous, bittersweet, a bit strawberry-like	Sinuses, throat, lungs	Expectorant, astringent, antibacterial, decongestant	Upper respiratory infections; drippy sinuses from colds or allergies; cleansing and toning upper respiratory pathways

Glossary

Adaptogen. Nourishes the adrenal glands and helps body adapt to physical, emotional, and psychological stress. Adaptogens include Siberian ginseng, *Panax* ginseng, reishi mushroom, and schisandra.

Alterative. Produces gradual beneficial change in body by cleansing, nourishing, and toning the tissues, glands, blood, and organ systems. Alteratives include red clover, nettles, sarsaparilla, dandelion, yellow dock root, burdock root, and alfalfa.

Anodyne. Soothes or relieves pain. Anodynes include St.-John's-wort, valerian, wild poppy, calendula, plantain, and rosemary.

Anthelmintic. Destroys or expels intestinal worms. Anthelmintics include wormwood, quassia chips, black walnut hulls, and garlic.

Antiemetic. Counteracts nausea and relieves vomiting. Antiemetics include peppermint, chamomile, fennel, and anise.

Antipyretic (febrifuge). Reduces fever. Antipyretics include elder flower, yarrow, rosemary, and lemon water.

Antiseptic. Destroys or inhibits pathogenic bacteria. Antiseptics include calendula, usnea, sage, echinacea, lemon, goldenseal, and myrrh.

Antispasmodic. Relieves or checks spasms or cramps. Antispasmodics include St.-John's-wort, rosemary, chamomile, and lavender.

Appetizer. Stimulates the appetite. Appetizers include gentian, ginger, angelica, cardamom, fennel, and Oregon grape root.

Aromatic. Has an agreeable odor and often stimulates digestion. Aromatics include mint, fennel, chamomile, lavender, and rosemary.

Astringent. Contracts tissue, reducing secretions and inflammation. Astringents include black tea, chamomile, yarrow, white oak bark, and comfrey leaf.

Carminative. Aids digestion and expels gas from the intestines. Carminatives include anise, fennel, peppermint, cardamom, ginger, cinnamon, and chamomile.

Cathartic (laxative). Empties the bowels. Cathartics include senna, coffee berry, cascara sagrada, and buckthorn bark.

Demulcent. Soothes, protects, and heals irritated tissue. Demulcents include plantain, chickweed, mullein, calendula, and self-heal.

Diaphoretic. Opens pores and promotes perspiration. Diaphoretics include elder flower, yarrow, peppermint, and ginger.

Diuretic. Increases the secretion and expulsion of urine. Diuretics include dandelion, nettle, parsley, burdock, and chickweed.

Emmenagogue. Promotes menstrual flow. Emmenagogues include angelica, ginger, blue/black cohosh, pennyroyal, and motherwort. These are contraindicated in pregnancy.

Emollient. Used externally to soften and soothe. Emollients include malva, calendula, borage, primrose, and violet flowers.

Expectorant. Loosens/expels mucus from respiratory passages. Expectorants include ginger, cayenne, yerba santa, and osha root.

Hemostatic. Stops bleeding. Hemostatics include yarrow, shepherd's purse, nettle, cayenne, and lemon balm.

Nervine. Calms, soothes and strengthens the nerves. Nervines include wild oat, St.-John's-wort, chamomile, and skullcap.

Purgative. Promotes vigorous emptying of the bowels. Purgatives include senna, buckthorn bark, coffee berry, and cascara sagrada.

Sedative. Soothing and quieting, reducing nervousness. Sedatives include wild lettuce, passionflower, valerian, chamomile, and hops.

Stimulant. Excites or quickens activity or physiological processes; usually contains caffeine. Stimulants include yerba mate, guarana, and green tea.

Tonic. Strengthens and invigorates specific organs or entire body. Tonics include nettle, red clover, wild oat, burdock, dandelion, codonopsis, schizondra, hawthorn, and ginseng.

Vulnerary. Soothes and heals the skin; useful herbs for salves and poultices. Vulneraries include calendula, chickweed, plantain, and St.-John's-wort.

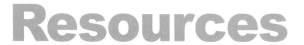

Resources

Herbs and Natural Products

Country Kitchen Herb Farm
5647 Cloud's Rest
Mariposa, CA 95338
(209) 742-6363
Call for information about tours and classes too. Great place to visit!

Dry Creek Herb Farm
13935 Dry Creek Road
Auburn, CA 95602
(530) 878-2441
Fax: (530) 878-6772

Frontier Herb Co-Op
P.O. Box 299
Norway, IA 53218
(800) 699-3275
Bulk herbs and many essential oils.

Herb Network
P.O. Box 12937
Albuquerque, NM 97195
Fax: (505) 452-8615
E-mail: komara@unm.edu

Herb Pharm
Box 116
Williams, OR 97544
(800) 348-4344
Herbal tinctures and oils.

Herbs, Etc.
1345 Cerriollos Road
Santa Fe, NM 87501
(888) 694-3727
Daniel Gagnon's company: high-quality herbal extracts, bulk herbs, books, and more.

Humbolt Herbals
P.O. Box 574
Eureka, CA 95502
(707) 442-3541
Organic and wildcrafted bulk herbs, tinctures, oils, books, and herbal products.

Jean's Greens Herbal Tea Works
119 Sulphur Spring Road
Newport, NY 13416
(888) 845-8327
(315) 845-6500
Fax: (315) 845-6501
Web site: www.jeans greens.com
Fresh and dried organic and wildcrafted herbs; also containers, oils, and beeswax.

Monterey Bay Spice Company
719 Swift Street,
Suite 106
Santa Cruz, CA 95060
(831) 426-2808
(800) 500-6148
Fax: (831) 426-2792

Motherlove Herbal Company
P.O. Box 101
LaPorte, CO 80535
(970) 493-2892
Fax: (970) 224-4844
E-mail: mother@moth erlove.com
Website: www.moth erlove.com

Mountain Rose Herbs
85472 Dilley Lane
Eugene, OR 97405
(800) 879-3337
Website: www.mountain roseherbs.com
Bulk western herbs, herbal products, essential oils, jars, bottles, etc.

Pacific Botanicals
4350 Fish Hatchery Road
Grants Pass, OR 97527
(541) 479-7777
Fax: (503) 479-5271
High-quality fresh and dried herbs by the pound.

Sage Mountain Herb Products
General Delivery
Lake Elmore, VT 05657
(802) 888-7278
Rosemary Gladstar's company; check it out!

Sage Woman Herbs
406-B South 8th Street
Colorado Springs, CO
  80904
(719) 473-9702
Fax: (719) 473-8873
Website: www.sagewom-
  anherbs.com

**San Francisco Herb
and Natural Foods Co.**
P.O. Box 40704
San Francisco, CA 94140
(510) 547-6345
Fax: (510) 547-4234
Bulk herbs and oils.

**Simpler's Botanical
Company**
P.O. Box 2534
Sebastopol, CA 95473
(800) 652-7646
Fax: (707) 887-7570
E-mail: simplers@
  monitor.net
Web site: www.simplers.
  com
*Quality herbal extracts
and essential oils.*

Trinity Herbs
P.O. Box 1001
Graton, CA 95444
(707) 824-2040
Bulk herbs.

Wild Weeds
1302 Camp Weott Road
Ferndale, CA 95536
(707) 786 4906

Chinese Bulk Herbs

Mayway Corporation
1338 Mandela Parkway
Oakland, CA 94607
(510) 208-3113
Web site: www.mayway.
  com
*Chinese herbs and ready-
made products.*

East Earth Herbs
P.O. Box 2808
Eugene, OR 97402
(800) 827-HERB (4372)
*Reishi extracts and prod-
ucts, bulk herbs.*

East Earth Trade Winds
P.O. Box 493151
1714 Churn Creek Road
Redding, CA 96049-3151
(530) 223-2346 or
(800) 258-6878
Fax: (530) 223-0944
Web site: www.eastearth-
  trade.com
*Bulk Chinese herbs,
patent medicines, books,
and supplies.*

Shen Nong
(510) 849-0290
Fax: (510) 849-0291
Bulk Chinese herbs.

Spring Wind
2325 4th Street #6
Berkeley, CA 94710
(510) 849-1820
Web site: www.spring-
  wind.com
Wholesale to practitioners.

Herb Plants, Seeds, and Garden Supplies

**Abundant Life Seed
Foundation**
P.O. Box 772
Port Townsend, WA 98368
(206) 385-5660
Fax: (206) 385-7455

Elixir Farm Botanicals
General Delivery
Brixey, MO 65618
(417) 261-2393
E-mail: efb@aristotle.net
*Chinese medicinal and
indigenous seeds.*

**Exotic and Shamanic
Plants and Seeds Allies**
P.O. Box 2422
Sebastopol, CA 95473

**Horizon Herbs/
Richo Cech**
P.O. Box 69
Williams, OR 97544
(541) 846-6404
Seeds.

Richter's
357 Highway 47
Goodwood
Ontario, CANADA
L0C 1A0
905-640-6677
Fax: 905-640-6641
Web site: www.richters.
  com

Seeds of Change
P.O. Box 15700
Santa Fe, NM 87506-5700
(800) 957-3337 (catalog
  requests)
(888) 762-7333 (customer
  service)
Organic herb seeds.

**Shepherd's
Garden Seeds**
30 Irene Street
Torrington, CT 06790-
  6658
(860) 482-3638
*Herb and vegetable seeds;
many heirloom strains.*

Medicine-Making Supplies

Aaper Alcohol Company
P.O. Box 339
Shelbyville, KY 40065
(502) 633-0650
Ethanol.

Pharmco Products Inc.
58 Vale Road
Brookfield, CT 06804-3967
203-740-3471
Fax: 203-740-3481
Ethanol.

Sunburst Bottle Company
5710 Auburn Blvd. #7
Sacramento, CA 95841
(916) 348-5576
Fax: (916) 348-3803
E-mail: sunburst@cwo.com
Web site: www.sunburstbottle.com

Educational Resources

American Herbalists Guild (AHG)
Box 746555
Arvada, CO 80006

American Herb Association (AHA)
P.O. Box 1673
Nevada City, CA 95959

Botanic Adventures
P.O. Box 12
Soquel, CA 95073
(831) 425-FERN (3376)
Web site: www.botanicadventures.com
Jeanine Pollak's Botanic Adventures offers seasonal herbal classes, hikes, and overnight wilderness trips.

The California School of Herbal Studies
P.O. Box 39
Forestville, CA 95436
(707) 887-7457
Started by Rosemary Gladstar in 1982, now run by James Green.

HerbalGram
P.O. Box 201660
Austin, TX 78720
Excellent quarterly publication, well researched.

Herb Research Foundation
1007 Pearl Street
Boulder, CO 80302

Living Awareness Institute
P.O. Box 5381
Vaccaville, CA 95696
(707) 446-1290
Web site: www.livingawareness.com
Kami McBride's school offers extensive herbal classes, herb walks, and women's herbal apprenticeship programs.

Sage Mountain Retreat Center and Botanical Sanctuary
P.O. Box 420
East Barre, VT 05649
Apprentice programs and classes with Rosemary Gladstar and other well-known herbalists.

The Science and Art of Herbalism:
Rosemary Gladstar's Correspondence Course
P.O. Box 420
East Barre, VT 05649
Rosemary's joyful and inspiring course.

United Plant Savers
P.O. Box 420
East Barre, VT 05649

Health Institutes

The Cerio Institute
P.O. Box 65
Soquel, CA 95073
(831) 475-5472
Started by Donna C. Cerio, the Cerio Institute offers high-quality, comprehensive alternative health care.

Esalen Institute
Highway 1
Big Sur, CA 93940
(831) 667-3000
Esalen offers weekend and week-long workshops in massage, health, and personal growth.

Index

Note. Page numbers in *italics* refer to photographs; those in **boldface** refer to tables.

Other Storey Books You Will Enjoy

Herbal Teas: 101 Nourishing Blends for Daily Health and Vitality, by Kathleen Brown, with recipes by Jeanine Pollak. This guide to blending and brewing healthful herb teas features anecdotes from several renowned herbalists and simple recipes for the head and throat, digestion, nervous system, lungs, bones and joints, circulatory system, and more. 160 pages. Paperback. ISBN 1-58017-099-4.

The Herbal Home Remedy Book, by Joyce A. Wardwell. Readers will discover how to use 25 common herbs to make simple remedies. Native American legends and folklore are also included. 176 pages. Paperback. ISBN 1-58017-016-1.

Herbal Remedy Gardens, by Dorie Byers. Using simple organic gardening techniques, anyone can grow a healing garden. Readers will also find recipes, tips for using medicinal herbs, and plans for gardens customized to specific health requirements. 224 pages. Paperback. ISBN 1-58017-095-1.

Herbal Tea Gardens, by Marietta Marshall Marcin. This tea lover's gardening bible contains full instructions for growing and brewing tea herbs plus more than 100 recipes that make use of their healthful qualities. 192 pages. Paperback. ISBN 1-58017-106-0.

Rosemary Gladstar's Herbs for Longevity and Well-Being, by Rosemary Gladstar. An exploration of the life-extending properties of herbs such as ginkgo, ginseng, and echinacea and their use in cultures around the world. Includes ideas for healthy living and recipes to enhance the quality of life. 80 pages. Paperback. ISBN 1-58017-154-0.

Rosemary Gladstar's Herbs for Reducing Stress and Anxiety, by Rosemary Gladstar. Gladstar offers natural healing alternatives for common stress-related health problems, such as headaches, tension, muscle aches, insomnia, and depression. 96 pages. Paperback. ISBN 1-58017-155-9.

The Book of Green Tea, by Diana Rosen. This informative book explains where green tea grows, how it's processed, its history and lore, how to drink and cook with it, and how to use it for beauty and health purposes. 160 pages. Paperback. ISBN 1-58017-090-0.

Chai: The Spice Tea of India, by Diana Rosen. Author Diana Rosen uncovers the history of this "common people's drink" while providing recipes for making and cooking with chai and serving suggestions for tea celebrations. Readers will find variations on the classic chai, as well as information on the ayurvedic properties of its different ingredients. 160 pages. Paperback. ISBN 1-58017-166-4.

These books and other Storey books are available at your bookstore, farm store, or garden center, or directly from Storey Books, 210 MASS MoCA Way, North Adams, MA 01247, or by calling 800-441-5700. Or visit our Web site at www.storey.com.